Questioning the COVID Company Line:

Critical Thinking in Hysterical Times

Questioning the COVID Company Line:

Critical Thinking in Hysterical Times

Laurie Calhoun

The
LIBERTARIAN
INSTITUTE

Questioning the COVID Company Line:
Critical Thinking in Hysterical Times

Cover Design: TheBumperSticker.com

Published in the United States of America by

The Libertarian Institute
612 W. 34th St.
Austin, TX 78705

LibertarianInstitute.org

ISBN 13: 979-8-9884031-0-4

For my nieces and nephew:

Caitlin, Alex, and Aidan

Table of Contents

Introduction

Questions about what I have come to refer to as the "Coronapocalypse" began to surface in my mind in late February 2020, as the news about what was going on in China and Italy began to spread. At that time, I was located in Nadram, near Klagenfurt am Wörthersee, in Carinthia, Austria, where I ended up staying from January through May 2020.

It struck me as very odd when, on March 10, 2020, Harvard University notified all of its students that they were not to return to campus following the spring break but to go home. Ten days later, on March 20, 2020, President Donald Trump announced that U.S. borders would be closed to all nonessential traffic. Citizens located abroad were provided with a narrow window of opportunity during which to return. This, too, struck me as odd, given that the outbreak had occurred primarily in China and Europe up to that point. Trump's move was, predictably enough, followed by a domino effect of other countries slamming their borders abruptly shut, no doubt under the assumption that the U.S. government knew what it was doing. (I briefly entertained the possibility that Trump may have closed the borders because he thought that Harvard must have known what they were doing when they sent all of their students home.) Many of the countries remained closed for most of 2020, some throughout 2021 and 2022, and a few are still closed to this day.

When I observed the news coverage of hordes of people returning to the United States, crowded together for hours at the major airports in the days following Trump's announcement, I mused that, if any of them were not already infected by the "very contagious" virus before being herded like cattle for an entire day in a highly congested setting — a true "super-spreader event," if ever there were such a thing — they certainly would be by the time they left the airport. I was so puzzled by these measures, taken seemingly under advice from public health professionals, that I pondered the following hypothetical question: *If one wished to spread the virus to as many people throughout the United States as possible in the shortest amount of time, what would be the best way to do such a thing?* The answer, to my mind, was precisely what the authorities had done: send possibly exposed people out to all corners of the country, places where hardly any of the inhabitants would otherwise have had any contact with anyone from Europe or China. In the United States, and everywhere and simultaneously throughout the world, government authorities seemed to be casting about in their usual way to "Do something! Do anything!" in the face of this new crisis.

My own bout of COVID-19 lasted about six weeks, ending in April 2020. I was alone in a house in the middle of the woods of Austria, which was the perfect quarantine setting. I can therefore state unequivocally and with great confidence that I killed no one's grandparents. It took quite a bit longer than the average flu for this virus to be expunged from my system, but my bizarre crackly cough and state of extreme fatigue did eventually subside. I had never before suffered a flu lasting more than three weeks, and through my experience of this illness I came to understand why elderly and infirm people might not be able to shake the bug. It was considerably more tenacious and resilient than the germs I had encountered before. I would begin to feel better, but then the virus would circle back for another round, making me wonder whether it would ever go away. It struck me at the time as entirely conceivable that the virus I had survived was not like any other infection I had experienced before because it had been genetically modified and was the product of a laboratory.

During the first six months of the Coronapocalypse, scientists and doctors who dared to suggest that the virus may have been "gain-of-function," engineered by researchers and accidentally let loose from the laboratory in Wuhan, were roundly denounced as conspiracy theorists. I let the matter drop, given the seeming consensus among nearly everyone everywhere that the origin of "the novel coronavirus," as it was referred to at the time, was natural. All mainstream media fingers were pointed toward Wuhan's live animal market, where locals were known to buy the ingredients needed to produce dishes such as bat soup. Whatever may have happened, I knew that, with time, the truth would emerge. There was an origin, and it would be determined, sooner or later, using the methods of empirical science. As of May 2023, the matter is still under investigation, but I trust that it will be resolved through genomic analysis.

By the end of June 2020, I was still in Austria, but in the city of Vienna, having visited Innsbruck, Salzburg, and Graz during the first weeks of that month. I felt fortunate to be one of the few tourists in the country, as the borders were still sealed shut to nonessential traffic, while many of the museums had reopened and the mask requirements, except on public transport, had been dropped. Having never visited Vienna before, I blithely pranced around the top travel sites with no groups or tour buses anywhere in sight.

My July 1st flight from Vienna to Bristol (U.K.) was canceled, as was my back-up coach to London, giving me more time to enjoy Vienna nearly tourist-free, despite being there at what would normally have been the height of the tourist season. Three weeks later, I was finally on my way to Wales, although in order to get there I had to make a stop in Ireland to change planes, as the Austrian government had put the U.K. on its no-go list. Needless to say, I found the illogicality and dubious health pretext of what was going on perplexing, and all the more so as I witnessed what was happening in very different places all at about the same time.

Large circular stickers were placed all over the sidewalks and piers of even very small villages, telling pedestrians where to stand. Arrows on floors and walls, both inside and outside, indicated the direction in which any persons who dared to leave their homes were permitted to walk. Many people were wearing face masks, and nearly everyone began wearing them when they were made obligatory by law. In London, I was shocked to see large posters threatening fines of thousands of British pounds for being caught in a station, on a platform, or in a train without a piece of cloth or plastic covering one's nose and mouth.

Throughout my months in the U.K., having already survived COVID-19, I was not at all worried about either contracting or transmitting the disease. That's what full recovery from a nasty virus means: I fought the virus, and I won. My body was protected by the very antibodies and T-cells developed by my immune system to rid myself of the unwanted intruder. Eventually, however, despite my determination not to allow a virus which I had already survived to disrupt my life any further, it became prohibitively difficult for me to stay abroad. I finally threw in the towel when British Prime Minister Boris Johnson ordered a nationwide lockdown, which made it impossible for me to travel to visit any of my friends in England, Wales, or Scotland, at least not without breaking the law. Nor was it possible for me to stay in hotels, as they had all been forced to close. I flew back to the United States on November 16, 2020, and have spent the last two years exploring new places in my homeland while waiting for international restrictions to be lifted and borders to open again.

Amidst this upheaval in my peripatetic life, Scott Horton contacted me in July 2020 to invite me to contribute actively to the Libertarian Institute. I reasoned at the time that it might be a good thing for me to set down on paper my ideas about what was transpiring, which I proceeded to do. I ended up composing more than twenty essays treating various aspects of the Coronapocalypse, some of which were met with anger and even enmity from people whom I had formerly regarded as entirely rational friends and family members. But I would not be shouted to silence, for questions continued to surface in my mind. Indeed, as time progressed, I became more and more intrigued about how it was that the government had managed to forge near unanimity among much of the populace about any and every policy, even those which made absolutely no sense from an empirical science standpoint. The strangely seductive trope "Listen to The Science!" was parroted by people from all walks of life (often with no background in science, much less metascience) and became a ready-to-brandish rhetorical weapon used to dismiss out of hand anyone who dared to disagree with the COVID company line.

Together these writings chart my intellectual consternation throughout the two and a half years spanning this exceptional period of history. The essays collected in this volume represent the reflections of a critical mind in a time of mass hysteria. My intention in investigating a range of political and philosophical questions related to the COVID-19 outbreak, and the response of governments to it, was not to promote any particular program but, rather, to use reason to try to make sense of what I was witnessing.

I have included the date of the first publication of each of these essays, in addition to the place where it was written, and I present the writings in the order in which they appeared at LibertarianInstitute.org. Two of the chapters (Chapters 14 and 19) have been slightly augmented to make the connections to the COVID crisis clearer. Sources linked to the original essays have been verified and are provided as endnotes.

1. COVID-19 Controversies and Communitarianism

August 3, 2020
Pontyclun, Wales, U.K.

The ongoing controversies swirling about COVID-19 continue to confound me. Not the fact that questions have been posed and "conspiracies" rejected but, rather, that many parties on both sides of every COVID-19 divide — regarding lockdowns, masks, vaccines, whether children should go to school and healthy people should go to work, etc. — appear to be thoroughly convinced that the truth is on their side and that those who disagree with them are "nutcases." Of course, the same is true about most any dispute on social media today, but when it comes to COVID-19, the adherents to various "self-evident tenets" have achieved a new and more vicious degree of smug sanctimoniousness.

On the one hand, we have people who seem to be truly convinced that those who don masks are Jesus-like characters who engage in "radical acts of kindness," as one person on my Facebook timeline characterized them, including, apparently, herself. On the other hand, we have people who guffaw at the sight of face-masked persons sunbathing on a vast expanse of sandy beach or while driving all alone in their cars, windows rolled up. Surely there are facts, grounded in science, to consider, but proponents of masks are so convinced that "The Science" is on their side that they facilely (and fallaciously) slide between interpretations according to which those who refuse to wear masks are evil, selfish, stupid, and/or ignorant. Common sense would certainly seem to dictate that illnesses can be transmitted through saliva — is that not in fact why restaurants sterilize glassware and eating utensils? But the COVID-19 mask controversy was considerably exacerbated by the government's own mixed messages on the topic. Even pandemic guru Anthony Fauci appeared in an early 2020 YouTube clip stating that masks were unnecessary and mainly for show, serving to make people feel better psychologically. Later, after the video had already gone viral, Fauci's claim was clarified as an attempt to mitigate a PPE (Personal Protective Equipment) shortage among health professionals.

I am less interested in questions such as whether masks diminish the incidence of disease (obviously surgeons wear "surgical masks" to prevent sepsis in the persons into whom they slice), or whether molecules do in fact disperse and diffuse rapidly in open volumes of air (see Chemistry 101), than in why people are so vehement in their disagreement over whether and where masks should be required by law. From the beginning, the characterization of COVID-19 as a "pandemic" seems to have conjured in many people's minds images of wheelbarrows rolling through the neighborhood to collect corpses. (I suspect that to this day some people continue to check their bodies for oozing boils.) Nothing of the sort has of course occurred, and the risk of death to anyone under fifty years of age is lower than the risk of death associated with all sorts of activities in which we regularly engage.[1] No wonder young people are not worried. They are not being reckless at all when they go out with friends. Are they being "selfish," as the mask brigade maintains?

At one point I attempted to reason with some people on Facebook who were denouncing as "evil" (in a refrain reminiscent of ancient Greek tragedy) those who do not wear masks. Among other things, I observed that, in fact, contrary to the apparent beliefs of the pro-mask chorus, not everyone who does not wear a mask lives in the United States and worships Donald Trump, who famously "opted" not to wear a mask for months. This was met with a flurry of denunciatory responses, until I revealed that I myself had in fact been wearing a mask, at which point I became "evil, stupid, ignorant, and/or selfish" for entertaining the possibility that other people might hold slightly different beliefs. R.I.P., civil discourse in the twenty-first century world of social media. Alas, as virtual and physical reality converge, fueled by an amorphous blob of pseudo-information, fake news, propaganda memes, omissive charts, incommensurable data, and, above all, emotive outbursts, the verbal violence has been acted upon by some. Mask shaming in the States now takes the form of people attacking people who call out the unmasked and, for their part, mask wearers joining forces to shout people out of stores who dare to enter without what are regarded as appropriate prophylactic coverings.

I was in Austria for more than half of 2020, at the height of the Coronapocalypse, where the incidence of the virus has been quite low and the death toll still hovers just under 700. I know, I know: 700 dead people who need not have died, if only… (If only what? If all men were not mortal, perhaps?) Why was the situation so much less dire in Austria than in Italy, Spain, or France? My best guess is that the powers that be effectively locked down their elderly care facilities and did not, as New York Governor Andrew Cuomo did, send persons infected with COVID-19 into nursing homes to convalesce, thereby directly causing thousands of excess deaths. No one *intended* to kill those people, of course, but given the precedents in Italy and Spain, where healthcare workers proved to be the primary transmitters of the disease, having not been tested unless they exhibited symptoms, it seems not unreasonable to characterize Cuomo's action as negligent, at best.

Cuomo is not alone in having imposed government measures which will end by increasing the rate of death of some of the persons supposedly being protected. When for months hospitals refused to admit or treat any patients who did not exhibit acute COVID-19 symptoms, they were turning away thousands of persons with heart problems, minor strokes, and developing cancer, whose lives will end earlier than they might have, had they only received medical treatment in a timely way.[2] In other words, not all excess deaths recorded will be due to COVID-19 itself; some will have been caused by government policies implemented in response to the disease. Small wonder that the latest U.S. stimulus bill will contain broad immunity clauses preventing lawsuits regarding COVID-19.

In Austria, the situation seemed to be largely under control by June, at which point the mask requirement in indoor places was lifted, allowing me to travel throughout the country as a tourist without having to deal with the usual summer mobs, as places of business were open while the borders remained closed. Masks continued to be required on public transport, but it was plain to see by mid-June that many people in Vienna were not at all concerned about COVID-19, for they often stepped onto trains and trams with no mask anywhere near their face. They might take five minutes fumbling around finding their mask in their bag, then fumble around some more while getting their mask on. In some cases, they would then proceed to remove the mask in order to eat a piece of pizza or some other snack. They talked and laughed and sometimes coughed with their friends as they entered the closed space, often while munching, with no apparent recognition that the whole purpose of the mask requirement was to prevent their saliva from infecting fellow passengers with the dreaded disease. I must say that I find it somewhat amusing that there were three simple ways to evade the mask requirement in Austria while avoiding the risk of a 50-euro fine: always be eating; always be drinking; or, oddly enough, always be smoking. So a non-smoker could always get around the mask requirement by spending time in a smoking area. I'll leave that one for you to parse.

I also noticed that in the markets, museums, and shopping centers, almost no one actually observed the government's ongoing recommendation to adhere to social distancing, or *Abstand*, despite the brightly colored circles glued on the floor nearly everywhere to indicate how far people were supposed to be staying away from one another. (Does anyone have any idea where and how all of those circular floor stickers were produced and applied, apparently all over the world, during the lockdowns? Just curious.) I noticed the lack of adherence to social distancing guidelines especially on escalators, which are probably the easiest place to gauge whether people are making any attempt whatsoever to keep their distance, given that it is so straightforward to do in that case. I tend to mount an escalator two or three steps behind the person in front of me anyway, because I find it rude to breathe down someone's neck, but in the midst of the "global pandemic" said to necessitate the closure of all European borders, both internal and external, people were there, right behind me on the escalator, unmasked and breathing down my neck. The idea that such persons might be evil, stupid, ignorant, and/or selfish never crossed my mind. They simply did not believe that they were in any real danger or that they were endangering anyone else.

Even more strident than the "I am Jesus" mask wearers are those agitating for universal vaccination. This is another source of ongoing perplexity to me, as many of those who sing the praises of vaccines as the only solution to the crisis also vociferously maintain, sometimes in the very same breath (filtered through a mask), that herd immunity is not possible with COVID-19 because of its mutating quality. This is conclusively demonstrated, they say, by cases in South Korea, where recovered patients became ill again with COVID-19 later on down the line. So let me get this straight: herd immunity is not possible, but the bars in Massachusetts will remain closed until such time as an effective vaccine exists? (Is this some sort of sly backdoor route to reinstating Prohibition, I have to wonder?)

In pointing out that vaccines are in effect a fast-track to herd immunity, and so, if the latter is not possible, then the former is a pipe dream, I appear to have upset some people on Twitter, one of whom abruptly announced that he would no longer be continuing our discussion because he disagreed with my view on vaccines. *What?* Who knew that I had "a view" about vaccines? Is it really all or nothing? May I not express a modicum of skepticism about the prospects for a COVID-19 vaccine while simultaneously affirming that I am indeed glad that I got the Yellow Fever vaccine before going to Ghana (even though I was quite ill for about five days) because then, once in Africa, I knew that I was safe from the disease? No, apparently a person who raises questions about the feasibility of an experimental vaccine for dealing with a virus for which some claim herd immunity cannot be achieved must be categorically denounced as an anti-vax "nut case."

My aim was not to denounce the very idea of vaccines, but to make a much more modest, purely logical, claim: *not (p & not-p).* Either herd immunity is possible, in which case the surge in cases across the United States suggests that we are well on our way to achieving it, or it is impossible, in which case the prospects for an effective vaccine seem quite dim, no matter how many dozens of companies may be aggressively recruiting volunteers for experimental trials of what they hope to be the miracle eradicator of the dreaded disease.

In several contexts, I have heard seniors lashing out against "selfish" young people for congregating together in public places — at concerts, on beaches, in clubs and parks, and… *at work!* — which naturally raises yet another quandary in my skeptical mind. Who is being selfish here, really? My impression is that elderly persons, who are quite right to stay home in order to protect themselves, appear to misunderstand the nature of the world which they have created and are leaving behind for young people. What could be more selfish than to destroy the livelihoods of millennials who have been eking out their existence in what has become a piecemeal gig economy — with no house or pension anywhere in sight, and short-term contracts to earn just enough money to survive while whittling slowly away at their quasi-eternal student debt? If all of the people attempting to go back to work had neither rent payments nor student debt, then it might be reasonable to ask them to take even more time off. But when financial insecurity reaches the point where even having a roof over one's head becomes tentative, when the tent industry becomes a hot stock option, then that is where it seems time to draw the line.

To reiterate: those who are at a substantial risk of death from COVID-19 should, by all means, stay at home (which many of them do in fact own). They can freely decide for themselves whether visiting with young family members is worth the risk of being infected by the disease, given its specific targeting of advanced seniors. But how does preventing young people from living their lives offer any extra protection to those who are already in reclusion, terrified as they are (and, in some cases, rightly so) to step outside? Answer: it does not. If you are already disinfecting everything which comes your way and refusing entry to anyone into your home, then why should you care whether other people go back to school and return to work?

Now it does sound as though I am taking sides. But what I have concluded after a great deal of reflection is that the extreme measures taken by governments the world over to protect a tiny portion of the population fly in the face of the more general ethos of modern-day Western society. For better or for worse, we have found ourselves in a world where people are held responsible for their failures and given credit for their success. We do not live in a communitarian society, where economic equality is imposed and maintained by the state or by mutual agreement of the group. In our liberal capitalist society, when the government itself *prevents* people from succeeding, by making their only possible source of gainful employment illegal, then those people are doomed to fail, not due to their own moral flaws, but because they have been prohibited from doing what they would otherwise have done.

The untenable scenario in which young, healthy people have found themselves is what I take to be the best explanation for the magnitude and range of indiscriminately violent protests across the United States. People are not looting Chanel boutiques in search of bread or criminal justice. Rather, communities all across the United States are literally exploding under pressure. They have nothing to lose and so are striking out in outrage, not so much because of the murder of George Floyd — Why did these riots not happen, to this extent, in response to the many African Americans killed by police officers *before* George Floyd? — but in an expression of frustration and anger and, above all, fear about their uncertain future. Millions of persons (hundreds of thousands in California alone) are at serious risk of being evicted from their homes. While some states have implemented measures which will allow rent and mortgage payments to be postponed, they will have to be paid eventually, which means that those who were only barely getting by will not be able to catch up.

Whose interests matter most, in the end? When the advanced seniors with empty vacation properties decide to share their resources (in "acts of radical kindness") with the people being impoverished, and in some cases rendered homeless, as a result of government measures designed to protect those most vulnerable to COVID-19 at the expense of everyone else, then they will be practicing the communitarianism which they preach. I don't see that happening in my lifetime.

2. COVID-19 and Collateral Damage: Killing versus Letting Die

August 21, 2020
Nolton Haven, Wales, U.K.

The question of killing versus letting die has long been a source of puzzlement to me, particularly as it arises in rallies for so-called "humanitarian" wars abroad. Wealthy nations regularly "allow" people to die all over the world — of disease and starvation, as a result of natural disasters, etc. — so how, I have often wondered, does the professed desire to improve the lot of non-nationals serve to rationalize the dropping of massively destructive bombs upon their homelands?[3] Assuming the most charitable of all possible scenarios (as unrealistic as that may be), *even if* leaders have the best of intentions, some of the innocent people living in places being bombed will die as a direct result of the military intervention, not from the danger allegedly necessitating the use of deadly force abroad. Such deaths are written off as "collateral damage" and the policymakers thereby exonerated in the minds of nearly all of the people who paid for the bombing campaigns.

The case of COVID-19 has begun to raise the question of killing versus letting die, for some of the persons allegedly being protected by the government are being, or will be, killed not by the disease but by policies enacted to combat the disease. Notwithstanding the stentorian outcry of government interventionists thoroughly convinced of the necessity of lockdowns, closed borders, universal vaccination, and face masks, the situation is not at all black-and-white. Indeed, it is quite complex. Everything turns on the contentious concept of "preventable deaths."

The number one killer in the world, according to the WHO, is heart disease. No one chooses to die of a heart attack, but is heart disease a case of sometimes preventable death? Obesity is a major contributing factor to heart disease, so one might not unreasonably suppose that if people were permitted to eat only lean proteins, vegetables, and fruits, along with whole grains; if they were prevented from consuming fatty foods and highly processed, sugar-laden snacks with no nutritive content (beyond calories), then the incidence of death by heart disease would diminish. This could be accomplished most straightforwardly by outlawing the offending foods and imposing government-enforced portion control. No state has to date prohibited or limited the production and consumption of fried foods, ice cream, and doughnuts. Which is not, however, to say that no one has ever tried something along those lines. When former New York City Mayor Michael Bloomberg attempted to outlaw large volume sodas (defined by his administration as exceeding 16 ounces), the law was struck down as unconstitutional.[4] In free societies, it is up to individuals, not executives, to decide what and how much to eat, and whether the risk of dying of complications arising from obesity — not only heart disease but also diabetes and other problems — is worth the freedom to choose what to consume.

One meme circulating around the Internet shows a severely obese person in a mobility scooter wearing a mask and lashing out at a young, thin person for not wearing a mask. The meme is intended as a not-so-gentle reproach of those who created the negative health conditions which make them personally vulnerable to COVID-19. The insinuation is that severe lockdown and quarantine measures are problematic in a free society in part because some of the people vulnerable to COVID-19 have health-risk factors to which they themselves contributed. Obviously, no one should hold octogenarians and nonagenarians "morally responsible" for the age-induced fragility which makes them more likely to succumb to respiratory infections than are younger, hardier persons. But surely there are also some people who suffer from obesity, diabetes, and other risk factors for which they, too, are not fully responsible, given their backgrounds and, in some cases, genetic predispositions. Bad choices are bad choices, but when they are made in part because of how one was raised, say, by parents who made similarly bad choices (and going back perhaps generations…), then there is some cause for restraint in judgment.

On the flip side, some people should not wear masks — not only young children, but also persons with asthmatic and other respiratory conditions. While in the Dublin airport, where I had to fly in order to get to Wales (absurdly enough — because the Austrian government had decreed the United Kingdom a red zone), I noticed placards around the bathrooms pronouncing that "Not all disabilities are visible." The signs were most likely intended to prevent anyone from upbraiding persons using handicapped bathroom facilities who by all appearances are perfectly normal. But it applies now, too, to people who do not wear masks because of their pre-existing health conditions, to which only they and their doctors are privy. Angry mask-wearers who shout shoppers out of stores for not covering their faces simply assume that the "rascals" are not doing so because they are selfish or stupid (or evil or ignorant), when in at least some cases those people should not be wearing masks, because doing so would be more dangerous to them than is COVID-19.

No matter what people do, death by disease cannot be fully eradicated, but other categories of death would seem to be preventable. Take the obvious example of traffic accidents, which has been discussed quite a bit on social media in recent months. If there were no cars, then there would be no car accidents and, therefore, no fatal car accidents. Make driving illegal, and road traffic injuries, which account for more than a million deaths each year worldwide, would come to a screeching halt.[5] Despite knowing the risks involved, people choose to continue to drive vehicles. Despite the evident perils of motorcycles, which afford no protection in collisions with cars and trucks, people continue to choose to ride them. In some places, seat belts are required by law, and motorcyclists must wear helmets, on pain of punishment for refusal to comply. Yet there are people who ignore those laws, unconcerned as they are about the increased risk of death which they will thereby face, and knowing that they will likely be fined if they are caught. Those are the rogues, of course, but even some of the people who do wear seat belts and helmets will be killed in traffic accidents, not to mention the many pedestrians who endanger themselves every time they cross a street. These activities are inherently dangerous to greater or lesser extents, depending upon the place and population density, but rather than outlaw all personal vehicles everywhere, governments permit individuals to assume the risk involved in activities which may tragically end in their deaths.

New Zealand has been heralded by some as a "success story" in the global battle against COVID-19, for the country imposed a complete lockdown of residents and slammed its borders shut with the result that hardly anyone in the country has succumbed to the disease — as of August 19, 2020, the grand total of deaths ascribed to COVID-19 is twenty-two. This makes New Zealand an interesting case to consider in thinking about the analogy to fatal traffic accidents. I say this because, in recent years, debate has raged over fatal auto accidents in New Zealand caused by foreign drivers. Like COVID-19, such cases tend to command a great deal of media air time, contributing to the perception of grave danger to the people of New Zealand. In 2016, there were twenty-six fatal accidents in which foreign drivers appear to have been at fault, and by 2019 the total number of traffic fatalities approached 400. At least some of those deaths were caused by foreign drivers, even if the perceived danger is higher than the reality.

The government of New Zealand might have prevented at least some of the fatal accidents by placing a moratorium on non-national drivers, preventing them from renting cars and exacting severe penalties upon those who borrow cars from their friends and those residents who furnish cars to visitors. But this has never happened. Before COVID-19 (which we may in the future refer to as "B.C."), despite knowing that foreign drivers from places where traffic flows down the right-hand side of the street do occasionally drift over the line on the sometimes steep and windy roads of New Zealand, thereby directly causing head-on collisions culminating in preventable deaths, the government of that nation has, at least up until now, permitted foreigners to rent vehicles and drive, even while knowing that some Kiwis (New Zealand nationals) will die as a result.

Now, with the sudden appearance of COVID-19, most foreigners are no longer allowed to drive in New Zealand for the simple reason that they are no longer permitted to travel to New Zealand. There were no doubt visitors around when the borders closed, and some may have decided to hunker down and wait for the virus to go away, but the moratorium on new tourists means a sudden and significant reduction of foreigners renting cars and killing Kiwis in New Zealand. *Win-win!* Well, except for the thousands of poor souls who are now out of work because twenty-two people in New Zealand died of a virus. The thinking among the powers that be, of course, is that, if not for the severe lockdowns and restriction of liberties, many more people would have died there by now. Unfortunately, despite the refusal of Sweden to lockdown, we do not have as a test case any place where elderly care facilities were competently protected while the rest of the populace was allowed to roam free. Note, however, that Sweden's per capita COVID-19 death rate is still lower than that of some countries which did impose months of severe lockdowns.[6]

After the recent discovery of an outbreak of a few new cases (not *deaths*, mind you, but *cases*), the New Zealand government extended its lockdown of Auckland again and went one step further down a slippery slope, adopting as a national policy to force persons who test positive for COVID-19, along with their families, into quarantine camps. National elections have been postponed for a month as well. Authoritarian habits die hard, and one might surmise that once bureaucrats begin crunching the numbers of actual deaths caused in New Zealand by foreigners, they will eventually conclude that, if ever they are permitted to return there for vacations, they should not be permitted to drive. In reality, that would and could happen there — and, frankly, everywhere — if and only if all of the new COVID-19 czars had some sort of consistent principles and worldview, which, clearly, they do not.

For example, while in Austria for more than half of 2020, I was surprised to find that smokers were permitted to puff away in public places, even though it was impossible to do so while complying with the *Mund-Nasen-Schutz* (face mask) requirement imposed in response to the arrival of COVID-19. Apparently, then, it is fine with the Austrian government for people today to induce in themselves lung cancer in the years to come, while endangering other residents with both second-hand smoke and COVID-19 simultaneously. Healthy non-smokers not at significant risk of death from the virus, in contrast, are required by law to don face masks. If the risk aversion demonstrated by government bureaucrats in the face of COVID-19 were applied consistently, then cigarettes and personal automobiles would need to be altogether banned, in order to save people from themselves.

At first glance, smoking might seem to be a more straightforward case than obesity, for no one needs to smoke to survive, while all people must eat. Many human beings succumb to death by lung disease each year, usually as a result of having smoked. The dangers of smoking have been well-documented, and this information is now clearly printed on every pack of cigarettes, along with accompanying photos frightening enough to be screen shots from a horror film. Yet some people continue to choose to smoke, and many continue to die each year of lung cancer and emphysema induced or exacerbated by smoking. Who is ultimately responsible when citizens die such preventable deaths? Is it the manufacturers and distributors of cigarettes? Is it the government? Is it the voters who elect the government? Is it those who stand idly by watching others act in ways which endanger their own and, in some cases, other people's health? Or are not individuals themselves ultimately responsible for what they do and thereby become?

The truth is that we never really know how and why people became who they became, nor why they do what they do. This is equally true for those who choose to smoke, to overeat, to ride motorcycles without helmets, and to drive while intoxicated or on steep mountain roads overhanging cliffs even when the traffic rules are the opposite of those to which they are accustomed. Given the many complex factors involved in our choices, each one of which contributes to who we finally become, the default position is generally regarded as one of personal responsibility, at least in Western liberal societies, where people are free to drink themselves to destruction or to gamble their lives away in other ways, whether literally or figuratively.

Contradictions abound in the *Animal Farm*-esque world of COVID-19 because different government officials the world over, and within large countries such as the United States, have very different views on what is and is not reasonable to ask of citizens. Quarantine, border restrictions, and testing requirements have changed frequently, and it is difficult to resist the suspicion that much of what has been going on since the height of the crisis in the spring of 2020 is purely the result of opportunistic politicians' attempts to "Do something! Do anything!" so that they can take credit when the virus finally disappears.

In the current terror-tinged global pandemic milieu, where self-proclaimed "experts" are a dime a dozen, I continue to puzzle over why people are not simply being permitted to act on their own beliefs. Is that not the very basis of conscience? If anyone is truly terrified of being in the presence of unmasked persons, I would heartily exhort him to stay at home and to do all of his shopping online. Just as in the case of drunk drivers and motorcyclists with no helmets, there will always be people who do not do as they are told, or as you believe that they should. If you decide to interact with those people (for example, by driving), that is a choice which *you* make. To those who would protest that, in the case of COVID-19, many people are ignorant of the relevant scientific literature — or "The Science" — I would counter that the very same argument would lead to the conclusion that representative democracy should be abolished. Certainly, the manifest ignorance of both voters and elected officials in interpreting statistical data has become undeniable in recent months, with apparently intelligent people reading "death rates" of critically ill persons already in hospital intensive care units as applicable to the population at large.

Plato observed more than 2,000 years ago that democracy is the second worst form of government — after tyranny, which is the system under which an executive is free to issue arbitrary edicts at his own caprice. The last bulwark against tyranny today remains a republican constitution — and the insistence of some people to uphold that constitution. The clear and present danger is that of citizens who permit themselves to be transformed into subjects, which can be achieved through inducing a widespread fear of death — whether warranted by the facts or not.

In thinking about killing versus letting die, the case of COVID-19 is no less complicated than the cases of driving, eating, and smoking, all activities with built-in dangers and which are easy to abuse. Despite the strange, sudden, and surprising near-unanimity of federal governments worldwide in deciding to implement a range of draconian policies intended to save the lives of those vulnerable to the disease by restricting the liberty of everyone else, and prohibiting normal activities in which healthy people would otherwise engage, the unsavory truth is that governments are in fact increasing the risk of death for many people who are in nearly no danger of dying from the virus itself.

Among the more drastic policy measures implemented in response to the appearance of COVID-19 is that of restricting access to medical services for anyone who does not exhibit acute symptoms of the dreaded disease. In this way, the new virus has been given a much higher priority than notorious killers such as cancer, heart disease, stroke, and suicide. Hospitals all over the world have put "elective" surgeries on hold, postponed cancer treatment, and refused admission to anyone not clearly suffering from COVID-19. This is tantamount to claiming that death by COVID-19 is somehow worse than death by cancer, heart disease, stroke, or suicide. But why should anyone believe that to be the case? The answer appears to be that because COVID-19 has been labeled a global *pandemic*, it is supposed to be worse than every other cause of death taken together. The numbers tell quite a different story.

In Italy, the average age of persons said to have succumbed to COVID-19 has been about eighty. Many people in that age cohort die of the flu every year. Fewer people are dying of the flu in 2020, because some of them are dying, instead, of COVID-19. So the question is not whether death is fully preventable in all of those cases, for it is not. Sometimes one's number is just up. The question becomes, instead: Is the rate of death by *other causes* being significantly increased for *other* age cohorts as a result of efforts to prevent COVID-19 deaths in persons over seventy years of age? It will take some time to sort out the data, which is an ever-shifting sandcastle of poorly reported and misleadingly presented statistics. The United Kingdom, for example, recently reduced its official COVID-19 death toll from 46,000 to 41,000 when it was discovered that people who died of other causes but tested positive for the virus nearly a month earlier had been included in the tally.[7] In New York, critically ill patients sent from nursing homes to hospitals (where many died) were not counted as elderly care facility deaths.[8] In some hospitals, workers were instructed to write "COVID-19" on death reports, even when the patient had never been tested and may well have died of something else.[9]

Amidst all of this murkiness, one thing is clear: from the moment when COVID-19 was christened a *pandemic*, people have been conflating the effects of COVID-19 (illness and death from the disease) with the effects of government policies implemented in response to the disease. COVID-19 did not itself cause the collapse of the tourism and entertainment industries. Healthy people in those sectors stopped working not because they were ill or moribund but because their governments made it illegal for them to work. The mass unemployment around the globe of persons prohibited from working during the lockdowns — many of whom will not be returning to their jobs because they have been eliminated as businesses have either been permanently shuttered due to insolvency, or jumped on the fast-track to downsizing via automation — will have ramifying health effects, both physical and psychological, in some cases culminating in suicide.

Millions of people in the United States alone are at risk of homelessness as a result of having suddenly lost, through no fault of their own, their source of income. Homelessness will increase the risk of all forms of illness (including COVID-19), to which some of those persons would not otherwise have been vulnerable. Formerly healthy persons may succumb to alcoholism, excessive drug use, and other forms of bodily harm and disease as a direct result of no longer having adequate shelter. None of these effects will have been caused by COVID-19 but, rather, by government policies implemented in response to COVID-19. Will the government administrators who created the conditions resulting in excess deaths be held responsible for the sudden spike in suicides, the cancer deaths caused by late-detection, and the deaths from strokes and heart attacks which might have been treated? That seems unlikely, for politicians are busy appending immunity clauses to COVID-19 legislation underway.

When it comes to wars fought abroad, the populace tends to accept whatever their leaders say, so long as they profess to be acting with good intentions. We should expect, then, that the concept of "collateral damage" invoked so often in excusing the inexcusable, the annihilation of innocent people by self-proclaimed good-doers who kill rather than protect them, will be dusted off in the case of COVID-19. Death is death, at the end of the day, and the dead have no interest in the intentions of their killers. But "collateral damage" is a trope devised to absolve those who kill, under the assumption that good intentions wipe the moral slate clean. In this way, the policies being implemented to combat the new virus raise a much more general question about the power of governments to destroy the lives of people whom they claim to be protecting. Now, however, in contrast to bombing campaigns abroad, it's personal.

Why and how are governments being permitted to enact policies which endanger so many of their constituents in the name of the few? It's no longer just a barrel of "bad apple" cops who kill some of the very people who summon them for help or are walking unarmed down the street or fall asleep in parked cars. Millions of citizens in countries all over the world are experiencing an unprecedented level of insecurity caused by the very governments whose *raison d'être* it is to protect them. Tragically, the people who could and should be protected have not been (see the case of Governor Cuomo in the State of New York[10]), while those who never needed protection have had their lives upended, and some will die as a result. Citizens have no difficulty forgetting about the carnage committed in their name abroad, but what happens when the government wreaks massive havoc in the homeland? We are in the process of finding out.

3. Destroying the Village to Save It: Government Overreach in Fearful Times

September 23, 2020
Ragdale, England, U.K.

After months of lockdowns, border closures, and inconsistent injunctions issued by local authorities to protect some of their constituents by severely limiting everyone's freedom not only to move but also to act, and even to speak, the time has arrived for a robust discussion of the proper scope and role of government. The range of "emergency laws" being imposed by authorities all over the world in order to stem the tide of COVID-19, or to prevent so-called "second waves" of the illness in countries where it has already taken a steep toll, is amazing to behold. I imagine that more and more of these laws will be overturned in Western liberal democracies as lawsuits force judges soberly to confront the mountain of statistics being amassed. One hopes that they will find ways objectively to assess the real danger of the disease — relative to other common causes of death — rather than continue to permit government administrators to base their abrupt and arbitrary policy changes on scary-sounding "case surges," which have not been followed up by surges in deaths, thankfully. It is unclear to me why anyone would ever have worried about a second wave of deaths to begin with, given what we now know about the specific targeting of the disease, which at the outset the hard-hit Italians certainly did not. But, alas, fear acts as a powerful vise on the minds of even intelligent beings.

It is surprising that so much emphasis has been placed on cases, rather than deaths, because nearly everyone now does seem to know that many "infected" persons show only minor or no symptoms at all. The CDC itself included a text to that effect in all of its early reports on the new coronavirus, back when no one really understood what was going on, and it seemed a matter of simple prudence to do whatever "the experts" decreed. Hardly anyone seemed to wonder at the time why, if COVID-19 was a genuine pandemic, the CDC would be stating, almost in passing, that "most people" would not be adversely affected by it in the least. So is it a pandemic? Or is it not a pandemic? Here is the definition of pandemic in the Merriam-Webster dictionary:

> *pandemic*: an outbreak of a disease that occurs over a wide geographic area (such as multiple countries or continents) and typically affects a significant proportion of the population.

In war theaters, those running the show have always hedged their bets, and the same thing is happening today in the theater of COVID-19. *Better to err on the side of caution!* appears to be the thinking, as at least some politicians must have believed when in October 2002 they granted President George W. Bush the authority to wage war on Iraq whenever he pleased, with no further need to consult the legislature. Once war has already been waged, the citizenry tends to line up behind leaders in a show of solidarity, even when it becomes indisputable that they have no idea what they are doing, as in the cases of Vietnam, Iraq, Afghanistan, Libya, and Syria, to list only a few of the many catastrophes in recent U.S. military history. Sadly, the same seems to be true in the "war" on COVID-19, as some have characterized it, and not without reason.

When authoritarian measures are implemented in the name of national defense, we are right to examine whether those measures actually promote rather than undermine our own interests, as in the case of the twenty-year "War on Terror." The summary execution of U.S. citizens without indictment (much less trial) was carried out under the authority of President Barack Obama before the not-so-critical eyes of the populace, most of whom did not even blink. Mass surveillance of all U.S. citizens — and, indeed, anyone, anywhere in the world — was justified in the minds of government leaders because of the danger supposedly posed to "our way of life" by violent terrorist groups such as Al Qaeda and ISIS. "They hate us for our freedom" became an oft-parroted trope, despite the ample evidence that, in truth, they hate us for our bombs, which leaders continue to this day to lob, killing innocent people while disrupting and degrading societies in lands far away.

The ever-proliferating "emergency laws" penned in response to the COVID-19 virus reflect a similar sense of urgency among bureaucrats. When persons are swabbed and then effectively punished (quarantined) for having "failed" the COVID-19 test, some among them are understandably baffled. One anecdotal case among thousands is that of my uncle, who needed to have surgery for the removal of a painful kidney stone but was forced to wait two weeks as a result of his positive COVID-19 test, despite exhibiting no symptoms whatsoever of the dreaded disease and personally suffering only from his kidney problem. There are much worse cases, of course, which involve potentially fatal illnesses: cancer, stroke, heart attacks, and the like. Nevertheless, asymptomatic patients continue to be denied access to treatment until they have first survived a quarantine intended to protect other people from death.

Making matters worse, there appear to have been many instances of false positive tests for COVID-19. Indeed, by some estimates, a large proportion of those who test positive but do not exhibit symptoms are not even contagious.[11] A bit of inactive COVID-19 debris (or "dust," as it might be termed) may lead diagnosticians to red-flag patients who are not dangerous in the least. The testing of people varies from place to place, with local authorities determining not only who should be tested but also what the threshold test sensitivity should be. These judgments are made on the basis of whatever strikes them — in consultation with their local "experts" — as relevant at the time. All of this makes it very difficult to know what any of the case surge reports actually mean. Many of the abrupt increases in new cases are obviously accounted for by the implementation of robust testing programs, particularly in places where no or very little testing was being done before. Yet government administrators continue to craft new quarantine, lockdown, mask, and social distancing requirements based on "The Science," because they do not know what else to do. Border restrictions on people hailing from countries with unacceptably high infection rates (in England, the magic number is currently twenty or more cases per 100,000 inhabitants) continue to be used to prevent entire populations from entering other countries.[12] In this way, all people of such nations are being effectively punished as though everyone living there were infected.

The government of Spain, no doubt viewing itself as taking extra precautions to protect its population, has gone one step further, refusing entry even to Americans residing in so-called corridor countries (deemed safe) and who have not been in the United States since the crisis began. So what is the health pretext in that case supposed to be, exactly? It is also worth noting that the tit-for-tat restrictions being implemented by countries — where one slams down a quarantine requirement, and then the other follows suit, preserving reciprocity — would seem to be based purely on politics, not public health. It makes no sense whatsoever for a country with a higher rate of infection to bar entry of people from a country with a lower rate of infection, who, by coming, would lower the host country's rate of infection, would they not? No, I am afraid that the numbers do not bear this out, for any changes in infection rate would be on the magnitude of rounding errors. If in a given country twenty-one people out of 100,000 are COVID-19 positive, even assuming that they are contagious (which many may not be), then what is the probability that any one person on a 200-passenger plane originating from that country will be a carrier? I leave this calculation as an exercise for the reader.

Having recently watched a few pandemic movies (*Contagion*, *Outbreak*, *93 Days*...), I have come to suspect that the primary problem with the new COVID-19 czars is that they are basing their policies on such apocalyptic portrayals, under the assumption that a pandemic is a pandemic. It has become abundantly clear that many of these people are altogether devoid of basic statistical analysis and critical thinking skills. As a result, they are indeed hedging their bets by waving their "Science" flags, under the assumption that anything bad enough to be labeled a "pandemic" by the WHO could kill us all. Thus we have, on opposite sides of the planet, the prime minister of Australia and the governor of Michigan proclaiming that emergency measures will be necessary until such time as an effective vaccine is readily available. The hubris of such a pronouncement is awe-inspiring. These leaders seem to believe that by wishing hard enough and pouring enough resources into labs all over the world — *whatever it takes!* — we can and will eventually defeat *The Evil Enemy* with a manmade vaccine. Alas, reality does not always conform to our wishes, and hoping for a safe and effective vaccine is one thing, while developing and testing one is quite another. There have, in fact, been attempts in the past few decades to come up with vaccines against other coronavirus and SARS variants, with no success.[13]

The movies in which pandemics are *The Evil Enemy* present truly existential threats to humanity, unlike COVID-19, which specifically endangers the aged and the infirm (usually both at the same time). Proponents of lockdowns and severe restrictions of movement and activity are reacting to COVID-19 as though all persons have a 99% chance of dying if they become infected, when in fact that is much closer to their chance of surviving. So if COVID-19 is nothing like Ebola (which does kill nine out of ten people it infects), then why are policymakers acting as though it is?

Consider Victoria, Australia, where the government has imposed one of the strictest lockdowns on the planet in response to an outbreak of cases in Melbourne. The people in that city are living under martial law, with police storming the homes of "criminals" who "incite" illegal behavior by encouraging others to attend public gatherings in order to protest the lockdown, mask mandate, curfew, and social distancing requirements preventing them from living their lives with any semblance of normality. How did the Australian government know that people were "inciting" such "criminal" behavior? Because the "perpetrators" posted their views on Facebook.[14] In the United States, Northeastern University suspended eleven students for violating social distancing dictates by partying at a nearby hotel.[15] (Note: they were not on campus.) The recalcitrant students will not be refunded their tuition and fees, and are barred from returning for the year.

Some may protest that I am making trivial objections. "World travel is a luxury and a leisure activity. Better to stay home and play it safe than to die! College students do not need to party! They should stay in their rooms and hit the books, helping others to survive!" But many businesses have also been fined or shut down for violating an ever-mutating array of regulations and requirements. Small business owners and contract employees have suffered enormously through the lockdowns in places where they are ineligible for government assistance, and thousands of small businesses will never recover.[16] Perhaps it will seem impolite to point this out, but it is nonetheless true that the individuals laying down the new laws have salaries which will never be disrupted, no matter what they do. They will not be losing their jobs and will not be rendered homeless, no matter how long the lockdowns remain in place, and no matter how often the rules for businesses are changed.

As an indirect result of political measures implemented to combat COVID-19, suicides are on the rise (including among people who are retired),[17] and cancer deaths will soon be, too, thanks to severely restricted access to medical care especially during the first months of the crisis. Some of the measures taken by governments to combat the dreaded disease have *directly* ended rather than protected their citizens' lives. Consider the recent raid by Peruvian police of a Lima nightclub in violation of curfew and social distancing edicts. In the rush to leave the place rather than be arrested, thirteen people were stampeded to death.[18] Assuming that the people at nightclubs tend to be on the younger side, their chance of dying from COVID-19 is much less than 1%. There were about 120 people at the nightclub, more than 10% of whom are now dead.

Six months into the crisis, many of the multi-million dollar facilities constructed to accommodate the expected flood of critically ill patients have been shuttered, some having never been used. Nonetheless, many citizens seem to be thoroughly convinced that the extreme measures which continue to be implemented worldwide — even in places where much of the populace depends on tourism to survive — suffice to demonstrate that the danger is real. Just as in the case of war, the harsher the means being used, the more fervently the people paying those in charge to do whatever they decide to do come to believe. What is the alternative? To accept that one was completely and utterly duped? There is a lot of conspiracy-mongering going on, no doubt an effort to understand the massive, concerted, global apparatus erected to combat a disease less dangerous to most people than is the seasonal flu. Conspiracy theories have swept in to fill the epistemological void because, some are convinced, there must be some reason, some agenda, some plan ("Plandemic") devised by a cabal of evil and mercenary geniuses (think Dick Cheney, the consummate war entrepreneur) who stand to profit and gain control of the ignorant masses at the same time. Otherwise, none of this makes any sense.

Certainly, there are agents involved (Bill Gates, Anthony Fauci, the CEOs of pharma firms, et al.) who have self-interested financial motives to create, produce, and distribute 9 billion doses of a vaccine. Suppose, further, that COVID-19 mutates, making it impossible for a person's natural immune system to provide protection for more than a few months at a time. What if, like the common flu, COVID-19 presents new variants each year, and governments decide (as some have hinted) to require everyone everywhere to line up not only for flu shots but also the latest and greatest COVID-19 vaccine? As improbable as that may sound, the State of Massachusetts decreed in August 2020 (amidst a flurry of new "emergency laws") that all schoolchildren and university students (both undergraduate and graduate) are now required to have seasonal flu vaccinations.[19] This despite the fact that the CDC itself reports an efficacy rate of 19% for the 2019 vaccine (the five-year range is 19–48%).[20] Imagine, then, that this requirement were expanded to include a jab for flu and a jab for COVID-19 for everyone. That would obviously be the biggest Big Pharma coup of them all — far surpassing the medicalization of ordinary troubles to which human beings have always been susceptible and which, since the U.S. launch of Prozac in early 1988, have been increasingly addressed through the popping of psychotropic pills. The lockdowns alone are likely to cause a huge surge in patients seeking a bit of help from their doctors to allay anxiety and stress in this ever-more uncertain world, where it has become nearly impossible to make any long-term plans involving anything beyond the perimeters of one's own home. Or tent.

The reason why conspiracy theories are flourishing is not only that people have too much time on their hands and nowhere to go. The truth is that the experts do not agree. Some maintain that shielding children from all germs will make it difficult for them to develop sturdy immune systems; others deny that this is the case. Do lockdowns help, or do they not? (See Sweden and South Dakota.) Is herd immunity possible, or is it not? If it is not, then why would anyone hold out hope for a safe and effective vaccine to be developed, tested, produced, and distributed before the virus, of its own accord, turns into something else or runs out of steam? Does anyone truly believe that the virus is going to exhaust its source of elderly and infirm hosts and then mutate, in an unprecedented display of viral intelligence, to target toddlers? In a climate of fear stoked over many months, *The Evil Enemy* comes to seem much bigger and more powerful than it is.

Once again, the case is not unlike recent foreign policy initiatives rationalized on the grounds that we must take the battle to the enemy before they have the chance to come to U.S. shores. I suppose that one positive consequence of COVID-19 is that nearly nobody fearmongers about terrorism anymore, as there is a new, bigger, badder bogeyman in town. Which is not, however, to say that the Middle East is not being bombed on a regular basis, just that even fewer journalists talk about it than before. In fact, there is not a lot of non-COVID-19 talk going on at all among media pundits. Across social media, people have already picked sides and spend their time denouncing as stupid anyone who happens to disagree. Again, this may have much to do with the fact that, having once invested in something, having been true believers, it becomes very difficult to admit error in the face of even overwhelming evidence to that effect. Politicians will continue to uphold their policies even as they destroy the lives of countless human beings. It happened in Vietnam, and it is happening today. To save the village, must it be destroyed?

There is no question that vulnerable people incapable of protecting themselves should be protected from COVID-19, because vulnerable people incapable of protecting themselves should always be protected by decent societies. But there are rational limits to the forms which that protection can take. Are terminally ill patients being helped by being denied the right to spend the last days and hours of their lives with their loved ones? Are independent seniors forced to live like recluses being helped by policies which prevent them from having any visitors? I think not.

What is being overlooked by policymakers is that there is much more at stake than simple existence. The "village" currently under siege is the social sphere. We are asked to wear masks, stay away from each other (no hugs or kisses!), avoid interacting with people beyond our "bubble," and not go anywhere unnecessarily. From the perspective of lockdown proponents, all of these measures are minor inconveniences in the face of a much worse consequence should we fail to comply: death. So we see children in schools wearing masks and sitting at Plexiglas-shielded desks to avoid the horror of anyone's tiny drop of spittle hitting anyone else in the eye. In fact, hardly any of those children would die, even if all of them were exposed.

"We will do anything necessary to prevent even one death!" proclaim some of the COVID-19 czars, apparently oblivious to the fact that human beings die all of the time. They want to protect the grandparents of the children, when in fact, the grandparents are perfectly capable of deciding what are and are not acceptable risks to themselves. For some, interacting with grandchildren is a primary source of joy. Being retired, they look forward to nothing more than spending time with their extended family. That is a choice which they can and should be able freely to make. And, lest we forget, children are vulnerable, too, not to the dreaded disease, but to the climate of fear in which they are currently being raised. Schoolchildren forced to wear masks do not see their peers' smiles and frowns, and hear only their muffled words and laughs. Some of them may avoid socializing altogether because it has become not only so strange but also prohibitively difficult to do. They have less reason than ever before for putting their iPhones away.

Before COVID-19, people who washed their hands a hundred times a day and avoided contact with others for fear of contracting diseases were diagnosed as germophobes suffering from Obsessive Compulsive Disorder (OCD). Human beings who scrupulously avoided social gatherings were said to suffer from social anxiety disorders. Now, however, social distancing requirements in venues as banal as grocery stores are causing people to behave as though their fellow shoppers were infected with the Black Plague. In some places, store clerks upbraid customers for violating one-way arrow requirements when they run back to pick up a forgotten carton of milk before returning to their place on one of the circular floor stickers at the checkout line. (Yes, that happened to me. Yes, I was wearing a mask.)

Many people have accepted all of the new restrictions on behavior as "the new normal," and two weeks of this sort of thing may not cause lasting harm to anyone. Six months, however, is a significant portion of a child's life, and we have experts today forecasting that emergency measures will persist well into 2021 or beyond. But should the existence of a virus, which may or may not ever go away, be used as the pretext for dictating how conscious, intelligent, free creatures should live?

4. The Intellectual Fraud of "Listen to The Science!"

October 23, 2020
Sheringham, England, U.K.

With the arrival of COVID-19 on the scene, many people have been seduced into believing that they must "Listen to The Science!" and do whatever the self-proclaimed experts tell them to do. That this is charlatanry, pure and simple, follows from the fact that science says absolutely nothing about what we should or should not do. Those are questions of value, answers to which are provided by intelligent, conscious, and sentient human beings who thereby advance a perspective and promote their own values. Waving a "Follow The Science" flag distinguishes one not as a person of superior intellect and moral constitution but as someone who is easily duped and slings slogans as a way of covering up a lack of understanding — specifically, of how empirical science actually works. To refuse to wave a "Science" flag in support of political policies put forth by persons with specific value-laden agendas does not mean that one is a Luddite or an ignoramus but that one in fact grasps the fundamentally skeptical nature of the scientific enterprise.

All of the ongoing clamor about "The Science" reminds me of what I observed while a graduate student in philosophy at Princeton University, where many of my peers seemed to believe that by specializing in areas such as philosophy of science or logic, they distinguished themselves as intellectually superior to those who wallowed in ethics or other forms of value theory. Having earned my undergraduate degree in biochemistry, conducted a good bit of research in organic chemistry, and taught chemistry at two different universities before pursuing graduate studies in philosophy, I was never vulnerable to the prevailing climate of *scientism* — the elevation of science as a form of religion — for I already knew what science could and could not do.

Science can tell you about the facts — not all of them at once, and not immediately, but over time, as data is amassed and theories are proposed and rejected or confirmed. Those facts are always tentative, mere hypotheses covering very specific and limited ranges of reality. A theory of physical chemistry, for example, tells one nothing about botany, for the two types of theory cover completely different strata and phenomena. What are believed to be scientific facts are always subject to disconfirmation as more data is accumulated over time and better theories emerge. Apparently recalcitrant data must be somehow explained away by the best confirmed current theory, and when that proves impossible to do, then the theory must, rationally speaking, be abandoned.

Scientists throughout history have clung religiously to their favorite theories (especially those devised by themselves), but eventually, as new generations of scientists emerge, older theories become amenable to revision and even wholesale rejection by researchers not religiously devoted to them. It is not easy to do such a thing because one risks offending the true believers, some of whom may wield extraordinary institutional power and will vehemently resist suggestions to the effect that they are wrong. No one wants to believe that he has devoted his entire professional career to the elaboration of a theory which was false all along.

Philosopher Thomas Kuhn wrote a gripping book, *The Structure of Scientific Revolutions* (1962), about the social and psychological dynamics involved in theory construction and testing, the nuts and bolts of the scientific enterprise, which, like it or not, is conducted by human beings, with all of their foibles. It seems safe to say that the COVID-19 cheerleaders for "The Science" have never read the work of Thomas Kuhn. To refuse to subject data to scrutiny, to decline to reevaluate initial hypotheses, naïvely accepting instead the prescriptions of select gurus on faith, even in the face of overwhelming evidence that they were wrong, is to succumb to the charlatanry of scientism, not to champion science.

Not everyone accepts Thomas Kuhn's rather derogatory depiction of how scientists operate; some prefer to uphold the image of scientists as supremely rational and objective analysts. But even if Kuhn's picture was an exaggeration — some would say a caricature — even supposing that scientific hypothesis testing were some sort of supremely rational and objective endeavor, what could even the best confirmed and most widely accepted theories of science tell us about what we ought to do? The answer is: absolutely nothing. For a scientific theory's having survived intact over a reasonable period of time does not alone dictate anything whatsoever about human action. To suggest otherwise is to commit what is known in philosophy as "the *is-ought* fallacy," usually credited to David Hume, an eighteenth-century Scottish philosopher with a skeptical bent.

Facts are one thing; normative prescriptions for action are quite another. People blinded by science — who, I have noticed, tend to be those with no higher education in science — those who, like Milgram's unwitting experimental subjects, accept the decrees of men in white lab coats and decline to examine the values and interests being promoted by them, have simply been duped.[21] A most stunning aspect of this intellectual submission (which has analogues in foreign policy as well) is when subjects are persuaded to believe that conflict of interest is somehow impossible among scientists, despite being possible in every other realm. Why are scientists supposed to be untainted by worldly temptation? *Because they are scientists!* As though human beings did not *choose* to become scientists.

To see the distinction between the deliverances of science and the promotion of values, consider one example of a fact widely considered to be true, based on many decades of data collection. Science tells us that smoking will greatly increase the chances of one's dying prematurely. One's decision of whether to smoke or not, however, depends on one's values. If you find the pleasure of smoking great enough, then you may simply not care today that at the terminus of your life some number of years will likely have been shaved off as a result of your insistence on smoking. (No guarantee, of course. There are examples of chain-smokers who somehow beat the odds to become nonagenarians or even centenarians.) All things considered, you are much more likely to die of a lung-related illness if you smoke than if you do not. In fact, all activities in which human beings engage involve risks along with benefits. Each individual must make his own choices for his own life about which benefits do and do not outweigh the risks incurred in doing those things — driving, drinking, rock climbing, flying, scuba diving, traveling to countries where violent crime is prevalent — the list goes on and on.

What has happened in 2020 is that a few COVID-19 policymakers have decided for all of humanity that the risk of dying from COVID-19 outweighs all other considerations about what we ought to do. This is a value judgment, pure and simple, and yet it has been fobbed off as some sort of "expert" wisdom. Those who crafted the initial responses to the virus, beginning with the very labeling of COVID-19 as a *pandemic*, have rallied the "Listen to The Science!" troops for many months, with the result that their stance has become very difficult to challenge. Few of them seem capable of assessing the new data and revising their theory as the scientific method would require.

Despite adamantly claiming that they "Listen to The Science!" they fail altogether to recognize that science is not a static, eternal totem, but a method used to marshal a dynamic, metamorphosing body of hypotheses. The irony, of course, is that the most vociferous denouncers of anyone who questions the gospel are conducting themselves in the manner of religious fanatics incapable of admitting that mistakes may have been made.

Thus we find that without any evidence whatsoever for the efficacy of lockdowns, and in fact a recent pronouncement by the WHO that lockdowns have side effects which vastly outweigh any alleged benefits,[22] the lockdowns of Western states, along with border restrictions and quarantine requirements, continue on, with local authorities tweaking their policies only slightly whenever they decide that the latest "case" tally is too high. No matter that different kinds of tests are administered differently and to different groups in different places. No matter that the very accuracy of the tests has been impugned. No matter that there is no other example of a respiratory disease (to my knowledge) for which one may repeatedly test positive as "infected" while manifesting no symptoms whatsoever. No matter that cases in younger persons are rarely fatal, yet serial, obligatory testing of college students continues on. The COVID-19 gurus have decided that a case is a case. None of the death data matters because these people, who never understood the scientific method in the first place, much less the fact-value dichotomy, continue to claim that "The Science" is on their side and that those who disagree are selfish and illiterate ignoramuses. In the United States, the people of California, Michigan, Massachusetts, and other states have had to endure severe restrictions of their liberty and much economic hardship for eight months, with no end in sight. Across the pond, both Wales and Ireland, along with various counties in England, recently re-imposed strict lockdowns as a form of "circuit breaker" after surges of cases in some places where no or nearly no new COVID-19 deaths had been reported.[23]

Proclaiming that we must "Listen to The Science!" has become the worst type of virtue signaling on the part of people many of whom have nothing to lose from the lockdowns, given that their own financial security is immune to whatever policies may be imposed. Shutting down the hospitality and tourism sectors of entire cities, counties, and countries causes untold harm to anyone working in the gig economy, and yet the victims are themselves portrayed as immoral for refusing to sing along with the cheery refrain,

"We're all in this together!" Few among the populace have been able to press these points effectively, because the media and tech industries have overwhelmingly joined forces with the COVID-19 policymakers, promoting The Science™ company line while silencing those who demur. Needless to say, there is nothing more unscientific than censorship, for the scientific enterprise requires a continual reassessment of the facts. When new hypotheses are forbidden because they conflict with what one believes to be true, then science has come to a screeching halt.

Even more devastating than the effects in Europe, Britain, and the United States are the same policies enacted in less-developed countries by leaders who emulate Western politicians religiously committed to their initial responses. The same lockdown and quarantine "strategies" have been implemented in places where they could never, even in principle, diminish the incidence of COVID-19 death, even if it were true — which is not supported by data — that lockdowns worked in the West.[24] In countries where large populations live extremely close to one another in open-air shanty towns — places such as Brazil, South Africa, Kenya, India, and many other countries as well — there is no chance that staying in one's hut is going to prevent transmission of the dreaded disease. Meanwhile, police have ended the lives of persons in violation of emergency laws which in no way serve the people's interests.[25] But to understand how absurd it is to impose curfews and quarantine requirements on the residents of shared outdoor space, one would have to be familiar with basic concepts of molecular entropy, which we know from the many closed beaches and outdoor mask requirements in the West are altogether beyond the capacity of the COVID-19 gurus to comprehend.

Perhaps the grandest irony of all is that, by focusing exclusively on the hope of minimizing the deaths of the small percentage of the population vulnerable to the dreaded disease, the medical professionals who have been advising the COVID-19 policymakers have violated the most sacred oath of physicians: *Do No Harm.* Lockdown policies have harmed every person whose risk of death by other causes has been increased by preventing them from doing whatever they would have done, left to their own devices: working, visiting the doctor, and engaging in normal social activities which make life worthwhile, including interacting with family and friends.

With regard to scarce resources and policies which affect entire populations, science is silent about who should and should not be saved.

Should limited health resources be dedicated to the mass testing of young people not at serious risk from COVID-19? Should healthy children at nearly no risk of death be used in experimental vaccine trials? These are value judgments about which science has nothing to say. Anyone who suggests otherwise is a shyster or confused, and anyone who believes that men in white lab coats should be the ones to answer such questions has been fooled.

5. Beware the Nurse Ratched State

December 6, 2020
Abington, Pennsylvania

Advocates of minimal government have often warned against the "Nanny State," which rears its ugly head whenever bureaucrats try to tell people what they should do and how they should live. There is a sense in which all governments do that, through the very enactment of laws, but Nanny-leaders mete out prescriptions which vastly exceed what can be fairly portrayed as an attempt to protect people from one another. An extreme example of this sort of overreach occurred in the United States during the Prohibition era, with catastrophic consequences. Not only did outlawing the enjoyment of alcohol not prevent people from drinking, but it actually catalyzed a massive expansion of organized crime all over the United States, as career criminals stepped in to provide people with the means needed to imbibe. No one wants to go to prison, which is why murder was on the rise throughout Prohibition, with blood flowing in some cities nearly as freely as whiskey and wine.

Such unintended consequences have arisen wherever recreational drugs have been outlawed, and experiments such as the one in Portugal,[26] where drug-related deaths diminished significantly after decriminalization, may have helped to propel some in the United States to accept the legalization of marijuana. The State of Oregon recently went even further, by legalizing the possession of small amounts of hard drugs as well.[27] Just as economics played a major role in putting an end to the thirteen-year Prohibition fiasco, the voters of some states may have been persuaded to permit recreational drug use after having seen the massive tax revenues being collected through pot shop sales in states such as Colorado. Whatever the reasons may have been, the slow dismantling of the legal framework undergirding the "War on Drugs" is certainly a welcome development to anyone who rejects the Nanny State.

The trend toward tolerating alternative lifestyles more generally, however, conflicts starkly with what else has been going on in 2020, coincidentally one century after the ratification of the Volstead Act. Policymakers attempting to save people from COVID-19 have pulled out all the stops — going above and beyond, in their view — to protect their constituents by issuing new and ever-changing edicts about how people ought to behave. This might be more tolerable if there were any genuine benevolence on display. Instead, what we are witnessing is an increasingly despicable effort to blame citizens for the failure of policies implemented in response to the arrival of the virus on the scene. When restrictions intended to stop the virus are imposed but cases and deaths then increase rather than diminish, this has been taken to prove to those crafting the new rules that citizens did not in fact do as they were told, and they are, therefore, responsible for the current state of the health crisis.

I have been in Austria, Wales, England, and the United States over the course of 2020, and in each of these countries I was surprised to find the very same finger-wagging reproach of citizens by government administrators who wish to blame what is manifestly nobody's fault on somebody else. All over social media, angry mobs continue to lash out at those who refuse to stay home or "mask up," and many government leaders now address their constituents as though they were toddlers or, perhaps more aptly, the residents of Nurse Ratched's ward.

This is a strange conception of government, according to which politicians do not work for the people who pay their salaries but instead are their guardians, who alone can decide what the populace may and may not do. The phenomenon is not unique to the dictators-in-waiting who run states such as California and Michigan. Citizens all over the world are continually being threatened by government officials that, if the case numbers do not go down, then lockdowns will be ordered or tightened, and more businesses will be closed, and further restrictions imposed, as though anything anyone does at this point has an effect upon a virus which is nearly everywhere and beyond anyone's means to control. This punitive paradigm may have been possible to uphold with a straight face until late October 2020, and many on the cacophonous COVID-19 caravan in the U.S. and in the U.K. have ceaselessly carped about their own incompetent government's response, contrasting it to the approaches of the admirable leaders of countries in the European Union and Oceania, who obviously knew what they were doing!

But then along came the resurgence of cases in Europe, particularly in countries which had been held up for months as shining examples of how a government ought to manage the crisis.[28] Germany had tough lockdowns, mask requirements, and probably the best contact-tracing program around. They restricted the entry of people from any country with an unacceptably high "infection rate" (scare quotes are necessary given the widely acknowledged problems with the PCR tests[29]), and anyone at the border who did not present proof of not being COVID-19 positive was either quarantined or turned away (some were also fined). So how does one explain the new wave of "infections" all across Europe? It must be the case that the naughty plebeian Europeans were lying about their contacts, meeting in large gatherings, and brazenly violating social distancing and mask ordinances. None of the case surges throughout the Northern Hemisphere has anything whatsoever to do with the fact that more people invariably fall ill with the onset of winter.

In the U.K., Prime Minister Boris Johnson issued in November 2020 a nationwide month-long lockdown order in response to a resurgence of cases which villagers tended to blame on the haughty Londoners — who obviously had been flouting the rules by partying and congregating in pubs and then spreading COVID-19 dust everywhere they went — from England to Wales to Ireland to Scotland, and back again! That was, however, not my impression. What I found upon my arrival in London at the end of October (before the new lockdown) were empty streets, shuttered stores, and restaurants and pubs with very few patrons. Realty signs were all around, and the place looked frankly like a ghost town. My train from Norfolk to London was nearly empty, as were all of the trains I took in the U.K. from July to November, when I finally decided to leave in exasperation at the abrupt and arbitrary cancellation and closing of anything and everything I might want to do and see.

Throughout this crisis, not only the governors of Democratic states in the U.S. but also the prime minister of Australia and the health minister of the U.K. have exemplified the Nurse Ratched mode of governance, repeatedly threatening their constituents with ever-sterner measures should the epidemiological situation not improve, under the assumption that case surges decisively demonstrate not that the policy initiatives were worthless but that people were not following the rules. Sadly, many citizens, terrorized by the mainstream media's non-stop fearmongering about COVID-19, have accepted this absurd blame game, which has broadened what was already, long before March 2020, the chasm dividing a populace torn in two. Unfortunately, the situation is likely to get much worse, as those who blithely agree to do as they are told become increasingly intolerant of those who refuse to do the same. Yes, the small paper cups on trays will be coming your way soon. What will you do? People are already taking sides, and the ironies continue to multiply.

Leftists have often wielded the slogan "My Body, My Choice" in protesting any attempts by the government to limit a woman's right to obtain a safe abortion. It is highly ironic, then, that some among them should now be agitating vociferously for the universal vaccination of people worldwide against COVID-19. The "Listen to The Science!" crowd immediately shuts down all who dare to suggest that the decision about whether to allow foreign substances to be injected into their own bodies should remain the prerogative of those individuals themselves. They denounce anyone who resists the call to vaccination as "anti-vax," even when they are not vulnerable to the disease in question and have no problem whatsoever with time-tested vaccines. Those who express any hesitation whatsoever to roll up their sleeves are ridiculed as "anti-science," even when they are in fact scientists by profession. When none of those inflammatory insults work, there is always the tried-and-true "selfishness" charge: you are a selfish, heartless human being if you are not willing to vaccinate yourself to protect other people from death.

Let us look soberly at the scientific facts, setting to one side all possible conspiracy-mongering about 5G, microchips, the World Economic Forum's "Great Reset," chemtrails, or anything else. First, COVID-19 is highly contagious but nowhere near as deadly as the pandemics of the past, and it specifically targets elderly persons with other health problems. An overall greater than 99.5% survival rate is not the sort of danger which would ordinarily lead healthy young persons to undertake a risky regimen to protect themselves. Why "risky"? At the most fundamental level, because safe and effective vaccines have always required years to produce and test, invariably involving, as they do, unknown side effects. The reason for this can be summed up in a simple, undeniable phrase: human variability.

For any trait, sensitivity, capacity, etc., found in human beings, its distribution can be plotted over a bell curve with a tiny percentage of people occupying the extreme ends of the curve. Those people are the "outliers," who will be much more (or less) sensitive to a particular environmental factor than is the average person. Perhaps the simplest way of thinking about this human variability and its relevance to the vaccine issue is in terms of food allergies. People do not know whether they suffer from a peanut allergy, for example, until their bodies have encountered peanuts. Similarly, a person with Celiac disease discovers this fact only upon consuming gluten.

When vaccines are manufactured, they contain components with which a given person's body may never have come in contact before. Most people will not be harmed by any of the components, as the vaccines have been rigorously tested on other animals even before human trials begin. Once extensive, long-term testing in large groups of human subjects has been completed, then the company producing the vaccine can assert with confidence that the risk to patients is quite low. The risk is never zero, however, just as the risk incurred by doing anything whatsoever is never zero. There will always be some people who are more sensitive than others, and they may end up being harmed by one or another of the components of any vaccine. There is nothing mysterious or conspiratorial about any of this, and in fact it is precisely why vaccine manufacturers insist that, before distributing their product widely, they must be granted indemnity in the event of the unforeseen and unpredictable side effects upon a tiny percentage of those inoculated.

All of this to say: there is always risk involved in taking a pharmaceutical product. People decide for themselves, for example, whether or not they should take the seasonal flu shot, the reported efficacy of which has ranged from 19% to 48% over the past five years.[30] This implies, according to epidemiologists themselves (not "anti-vaxxers" or conspiracy theorists), that more than half of the people who have taken the flu shot have not been helped by the treatment in the least. Were any of them harmed? It is difficult to say, because people fall ill and die all of the time, and there are usually far too many variables working simultaneously to be able to single out the cause of post-treatment harm, particularly when the subjects are already elderly and frail. Those who sing the praises of the annual flu shot, including the public relations teams behind the aggressive marketing campaigns launched by governments to encourage their citizens to undergo injection, generally seem to believe that the efficacy rate is much higher than it is. From a consideration of the marketing material alone, one would be forgiven for concluding that the flu shot is rationally obligatory and 100% effective and safe. Having once examined the statistics, however, there is some cause for restraint.

Just as no one should be able to force you to drink green tea because *he* believes that it is good for *your* health, and no cancer victim can be compelled to undergo chemotherapy against his own will, individuals themselves must decide whether rolling up their sleeves for the annual flu shot is a good idea or not. Those who are young and hardy will most likely survive the flu in any case, and there is a real chance that the formula which they take — there are multiple versions every year — will not help to combat one or another of the virus strains which they happen to encounter anyway. It is literally a gamble. There are people who maintain that they never became sicker than after having taken a flu shot, but vaccine advocates quickly sweep in to silence them by insisting that they must have already been exposed to the flu before inoculation. In fact, the only reason for believing such an explanation is manifestly that one wishes to support the imposition of universal medical treatments. It may or may not be true. One thing is undeniable: pharmaceutical firms are profit-driven companies, whose revenues will wax or wane with general public sentiment about the benefits and harms of their many-splendored cures.

The current situation is quite a bit murkier than the case of the seasonal flu shot, because most of the COVID-19 vaccines being developed employ a novel RNA technology never before licensed for use in human beings.[31] In the vaccines which have stood the test of time (measles, polio, etc.), a tiny amount of pathogen protein is introduced into a patient's body so that it will preemptively ready itself for an immune response in the event that the virus is later encountered. Usually, the virus matter introduced is dead, but sometimes it is live, and this is by design — it depends on the pathogen and is determined through extensive experimentation. A live vaccine induces a minor bout of the disease, which is much less likely to lead to death than is an unprotected body's encounter with the wild virus. Anecdotally, I can report that after having received an obligatory Yellow Fever vaccine (which is live) before traveling to Ghana in 2008, I was quite ill for about five days. The cause and the effect were clear: I was suffering a minor bout of Yellow Fever, thanks to which my body developed the antibodies needed to protect me from the disease during my trip to Africa.

Suppose, now, that the new COVID-19 vaccines worked just as the time-tested vaccines do. In that case, before agreeing to be inoculated, a reasonable person would require some sort of assurance that the vaccine itself will be less likely to harm the patient than is the wild strain of the virus. Because the survival rate among people exposed to COVID-19 is greater than 99%, it would be prudent for a person to take the vaccine only if his prospects would be improved through vaccination. At this disease risk level, without any such guarantee, one may or may not wish to take an experimental vaccine. People in the vulnerable categories (especially advanced seniors) and those who are exposed regularly to the disease in healthcare contexts may well feel that it is worth the risk, and they will likely be first in line for the treatments once they are made available.

It is of utmost importance to bear in mind, however, that the vaccines currently regarded as most promising for controlling the outbreak of COVID-19 do not involve the time-tested approach. Rather than introducing proteins from the offending organism (or a simulacrum), the front-runner vaccines introduce foreign pieces of viral mRNA (messenger ribonucleic acid) which will instruct the person's own body to produce some of the immune system-galvanizing viral proteins itself. The presence of those pseudo-foreign proteins — coded for by foreign mRNA but produced within the human body — will then initiate the needed immune response. In other words, there is an extra step involved. The foreign mRNA is introduced, and then the person's body produces the proteins coded for by the snippets of mRNA, after which the needed antibodies will be generated by the body in response. This ingenious scheme (if it works!) involves the human body tricking itself into triggering an immune response by producing what are empirically indistinguishable from traces of the offending virus itself. What could go wrong?

Perhaps nothing will go wrong, but the fact (of science!) remains: such vaccines have never been used in human populations before. In attempting to discuss this matter with various people (civil discourse is not always possible with the "Listen to The Science!" crowd, ironically), I have been amazed that there should exist persons fully prepared to agree to totalitarian control over their very own bodies while knowing absolutely nothing about the history of vaccine development. They simply do not care that the novel vaccines are novel, or that those who volunteer to take part in the largest experimental trial of vaccines in human history are essentially offering their bodies up as Petri dishes to pharmaceutical firms. Some vaccine enthusiasts appear not even to know what mRNA is and attempt to discredit anyone who disagrees with their gurus in white lab coats (most of whom have financial ties to Big Pharma), despite the fact that plenty of published literature exists on the topic of vaccine harm. Advocates for forced universal vaccination appear to be unfazed by possible conflicts of interest and are not at all bothered by the sudden appearance of Bill Gates (whose company

Microsoft, lest we forget, violated anti-trust laws) in their social media timelines exhorting everyone everywhere to get on board with the global vaccination regime.

Beyond all of the factors relevant to new vaccines more generally, one can quite reasonably inquire, in this case, whether anyone should trust a company (AstraZeneca) which "accidentally" (through a "manufacturing error") gave thousands of its vaccine trial participants only half of their first dose, reported a 90% efficacy figure, but subsequently discovered that the true efficacy rate in those fully dosed was only about 62%. In other words, in the AstraZeneca trial in question, the less vaccine the subjects received, the better they fared.[32] None of this is to suggest that anyone should expect laboratory technicians to be perfect, for they are human. But that is part of the gamble one takes in agreeing to participate in such a study, as can be seen throughout the history of vaccine development, which has left many bodies in its wake, mostly animals of other species, but also some human beings.

The reason why the healthy Western subjects of pharmaceutical drug trials have always been generously remunerated — in the Third World they are not[33] — is that they are risking their own well-being and even life by agreeing to ingest substances with unknown side effects, which cannot be predicted *a priori*. Indemnity clauses are always included in the contracts for those who agree to participate in experimental drug trials precisely in order to prevent any victims (or their survivors) from seeking compensation should something go awry. It is of course possible, and one certainly hopes, that the injection of foreign mRNA into human bodies may not cause any lasting harm, but the unvarnished truth is that we simply do not know what the long-range and unforeseen consequences will be, because this has never been done before.

In all of the excitement over the splendid reported efficacy rates (90%, 94%, and over 95%) of the front-runners in the great COVID-19 vaccine race, I have seen no mention by anyone of the *survival* outcomes of placebo subject classes.[34] Why might that be? Whenever new drugs and remedies are scientifically tested, this is done with a contrast class of subjects who are given not the treatment being studied but a placebo substance considered to be inert *vis-à-vis* the disease to be defeated. This is the only way to demonstrate that the remedy is more helpful than doing nothing at all. In the case of COVID-19, there are a few key factors to bear in mind. First, based on the death charts of the CDC, the WHO, and many other institutions as well, it is evident that *any* placebo remedy which I myself decide to take — water, vegetables, vitamin C, quinine, even air — already has a 99.5% chance of keeping me alive, even if I am exposed to and become infected with COVID-19. I may, therefore, stick with the placebo for the entirely rational reason that its efficacy rate in keeping me alive is likely just as high, if not higher, than that of any possible vaccine.

Big Pharma's tactic of neglecting to report on the outcomes of placebo studies for its vast array of antidepressants and anxiety remedies was for years ignored. Eventually, a few courageous psychiatrists and psychologists revealed that, for many of the best-selling psych meds prescribed to millions of people all over the world, placebo subjects fared just as well and sometimes even better than those taking the drugs, particularly in long-range studies.[35] In other words, many people prescribed psychotropic medication for acute cases of depression, anxiety, and grief induced by life traumas such as the loss of a loved one would have improved over time, even if they had taken no drug at all. Mention of such results was routinely omitted from reports touting the efficacy of the new products for the plainly diaphanous reason that taking no medication does not produce any profit for drug manufacturers.

Similarly, the companies touting the virtues of their new vaccines designed to save humanity from COVID-19 make no mention of placebo class survival outcomes. Nonetheless, many people have been encouraged by the reported results, relieved that at last they will be able to get back to living their lives as they please. In reality, the current misery of healthy individuals being victimized not by COVID-19 but by political policies crafted in response to the virus has no logical connection to the invention or success of any vaccine. Rolling up one's sleeve cannot be made a condition upon ending policies which do not protect but rather harm most of humanity. (See Appendix A, the text of the Great Barrington Declaration.) Instead, the policies should be ended because they never had, and never will have, the advertised effects.[36]

When anyone dares to express skepticism about the decrees of the new COVID-19 czars, this is taken to illustrate that they need to be protected from themselves and also from harming others. Somehow, we have found ourselves in a world governed by Nurse Ratched-esque individuals who repeatedly scold us for the failure of their previous policies to put an end to COVID-19 and appear ready and willing to punish us further for not agreeing to do as they say and, now, to roll up our sleeves. They call it "treatment," and they have already purchased, using taxpayer funds (what else?), "free" vaccines for all. From the perverse perspective of these government officials, it is *our* fault that the virus is running rampant, and, therefore, we must line up for our paper cup on the tray. If any persons object to being made into the subjects of an experimental vaccine trial, for any of the many non-conspiratorial reasons outlined above, they are to be denounced as lunatic fringe extremists and deplatformed across social media.

This frightening transformation of citizens into subjects is now so widespread that even some business leaders are promoting the same line, apparently believing themselves to comply with what they have been told over and over again are the dictates of science. The CEO of Qantas Airways recently announced that they will be requiring proof of COVID-19 vaccination for anyone attempting to board their flights.[37] Needless to say, I will not be traveling to Australia again anytime soon, because my body is my own, and I do not agree to offer it up as a Petri dish in a large-scale clinical trial by any profit-driven company, and certainly not Big Pharma, whose amorality (at best) and manifest greed has already been firmly established through its many large-scale campaigns to drug everyone for anything — from infants to nonagenarians — with psych meds. (Did you know that "Prozac" for dogs and cats is now a thing?)

It is precisely because of the unavoidable dangers involved that individuals, who alone will bear any negative consequences arising from their choices, must retain control over what is done to their own bodies. Yes, there are COVID-19 outliers as well: younger persons who suffer worse health outcomes than the vast majority of their peers, and it is possible that any given person will be an outlier in that sense. But there are already mountains of demographic statistics available on the dangers of COVID-19, while none whatsoever exist yet for the new vaccines. Free people must therefore decide for themselves whether the risks of taking an experimental antidote to a disease are outweighed by its alleged benefits. When authoritarian leaders and their associates in the corporate world paint themselves as benevolent, insisting that they are only trying to save the world from the dreaded disease, they are forgetting the most important quality of their constituents and customers: they are free to determine their own destinies and to assume risks which they themselves regard as rational and to reject those which they do not.

The United States Supreme Court recently upheld citizens' First Amendment rights of religion and assembly,[38] even during a global pandemic, and one hopes that as lawsuits continue to wend their way up the judicial chain, the grip of authoritarian policymakers will be further diminished. Human beings should never be held hostage to the demands of those promoting universal vaccination, and least of all when their own danger of succumbing to the disease in question is small. If my own chances of dying from COVID-19 were 50%, rather than less than 0.5%, then it might well be rational for me to gamble, just as many cancer victims, out of desperation, have agreed to submit to experimental treatments. But I am neither sick nor particularly vulnerable to the novel COVID-19 virus, so I'll take my chances with my own immune system and my preferred placebo remedy of liberty. I may no longer be welcome in Australia, but there's always Brazil.[39] Or perhaps I'll go to Mars.[40]

6. Welcome to Zombie Pharm

December 23, 2020
Abington, Pennsylvania

Imagine a world where you were required to cover your face and nose whenever you stepped out of your home or when anyone came to your door. No one would know when you smiled or frowned, and the difficulty of communicating the ideas you attempted to share would eventually deter you from saying much of anything at all, frustrated as you would be by the annoyance of always having to repeat yourself. There would be no point in asking anyone questions requiring more than a "yes" or "no" answer, because more complicated replies would be muffled by their masks and not worth the time and effort needed to decipher.

Imagine a world where all inhabitants of a city, state, or country were told where they could go and what they could do, not only in public, but also in their homes and in privately owned businesses. Healthy persons would be quarantined to prevent other people from becoming ill. Good citizens would be enlisted and surveillance and tracking apps used to identify anyone who refused to abide by emergency lockdown and curfew orders or the required hygiene measures. Small business owners would be fined for attempting to run their businesses or for neglecting to enforce emergency laws. Employees would be arrested for attempting to go to work.

Imagine a world where private tech companies collaborated with government bureaucrats to censor your written speech. You would not be permitted to share texts which conflicted with the official story of whatever the authorities claimed that they had done and were doing and wanted you to believe. You could still write texts, on your own computer, but there would be nearly no one around to read what you had to say. The censors could not suppress texts faster than they could be written and shared, however, so some would slip through. This would necessitate visits from the state police to the homes of those who had attempted to incite violations of any emergency laws which happen to have been enacted by administrators to protect their constituents. Whether or not the measures actually helped anyone would be entirely beside the point, because everyone knows (from all of the "just wars" throughout history) that all that matter are the lawmakers' publicly professed intentions to do good. The perpetrators of what were deemed dangerous texts would be arrested and taken away, if necessary, by force.

Imagine a world where journalists were required to promote the official government line in order to keep their jobs. No text or report which reflected poorly on the military-industrial-congressional-media-academic-logistics-pharmaceutical-banking complex would be allowed. A few of those who "indulgently" refused to comply might then impudently begin their own publications, such as *The Intercept*, issuing their interpretation of what was going on in the few sequestered places (made difficult to find by Google) where independent journalism was still possible.

Imagine a world where the independent media, too, had been infiltrated by persons keen to hold the line, to defend what they had been persuaded to believe (by hook or by crook, carrots or sticks) must be upheld as the truth. Those who attempted to share inconvenient "disinformation" or "fake news," as it would be denounced, would then have their works edited to conform with "the official story." The "traitors," as they would be characterized, who disagreed would have two choices: either to stop writing or to flee to another place with even fewer readers than before, such as Substack.

Imagine a world where publishers who revealed crimes committed by governments would be subject to criminalization: arrest, incarceration, isolation, extradition, and more. Those who exposed murderous crimes would themselves be treated as though they were violent criminals, even when they had never in their lives wielded any implement of dissent beyond a pen.

Imagine a world where oppressive lockdown and curfew policies were said to be necessitated by case surges of "infections" in persons many of whom, while testing positive, manifested no symptoms at all. Suppose that the tests being used were revealed to be notoriously inaccurate, by some estimates, 90% inaccurate. Yet the testing continued on, ever faster and more furiously, and the case surges would serve as the basis for preventing healthy people from living their lives. When vaccines emerged, everyone who tested positive before but survived would still need to be inoculated, because, as the "Listen to The Science!" crowd would insist, it might be possible to become reinfected. People who had already survived the dreaded disease would only know that they were safe and not a menace to public health if they took the new vaccines, whatever they were, and whether or not they had been demonstrated to prevent and transmit infection, and no matter what the unknown side effects might be. Because, obviously: Science.

Imagine a world where people with life-threatening diseases were required to postpone their treatment because another disease, 95% of whose victims were octogenarians or older, had been designated by select "expert" epidemiologists as more dangerous and life-threatening than cancer, heart disease, stroke, and the other top killers of human beings.

Imagine a world where distraught and desperate people reduced to poverty and rendered homeless through not being permitted to work began turning to deadly drugs such as heroin, sometimes fentanyl-laced, with the result that, in some cities (such as San Francisco), more persons died of overdoses than of the disease serving as the pretext for the laws forbidding those people from working.

Imagine a world where citizens were required to undergo medical treatments not known to prevent disease but believed to alleviate the symptoms of a disease for which the vast majority of humanity suffer only minor symptoms. This would be undertaken in the name of public health, but the effect would be to harm some of those who were not vulnerable to the disease and essentially had been tricked or coerced — since uninformed "consent" is not really consent — into volunteering as subjects in an enormous experimental trial with the aim of determining the outcome of introducing into human bodies certain foreign substances deemed potentially profitable by the companies which produced them. Most people would line up enthusiastically for such vaccines on the basis of widely disseminated claims of 90% and 95% efficacy lauded by well-respected experts, with details about the "known unknowns" and "unknown unknowns" available only in the fine print of a few more nuanced articles, which nearly no one read.

Imagine a world where people who had already survived the dreaded disease and had also been vaccinated were nonetheless required to abide by all of the ongoing hygiene measures, from wearing a mask, to staying home, to taking more vaccines on a schedule determined by their government. There would be no need to explain what any of this was for because all good citizens would already be accustomed to reciting the mumbled refrains (behind their masks): "Extraordinary times call for extraordinary measures!" and "We're all in this together!" Everyone would have to comply; everyone would need to be quiet; everyone would be required by law to roll up his sleeve for the clearly compelling reason that a global pandemic was tearing through the world like a tsunami, wiping out everyone in its path. Except that most of the victims were dying at the same rate and age as the actuary tables would have predicted even if the culprit virus had never arrived on the scene. And the death toll over the course of the year would be about the same as for any other year, but with a slightly different distribution in causes of death.

Imagine a world where you were required to present your health record on demand and you would not be permitted to enter stores, restaurants, schools, to work, or to travel without first proving that you had agreed to participate in an experimental vaccine trial for a disease from which you were at minimal risk of harm. The local health authorities would determine when you needed to present yourself again for a new treatment, as the virus in question could morph unpredictably over short intervals of time into something else, thus necessitating that you and everyone else on the planet prepare your bodies once again, just in case this time around it might be more dangerous to you and those around you.

Imagine a world where a healthy person's refusal to undergo medical treatment for a potential future possible disease to which he was not vulnerable, according to all available statistical indicators, was taken as proof of his suffering from another disease, Oppositional Defiant Disorder (ODD), as clearly indicated in the latest edition of the *Diagnostic Statistical Manual of Mental Disorders* (*DSM*). The person thus diagnosed would be required by law to submit to whatever medication would make him more amenable to the other forms of medical treatment to which he was opposed because obviously there would be something very wrong with him, constituting as he would a grave danger to public health.

Imagine a world in which children were taught from an early age that it was unsafe to touch other human beings or to be touched by them. They would be required to wear masks and full-face plastic shields and to wash their hands frequently and to attend school by video conference because, they would be sternly instructed, otherwise they might kill somebody else's parents or grandparents, even though they themselves were not ill. If the children found any of this a source of anxiety, they would be prescribed psychiatric medications to transform their view of the world, so that they would accept rather than reject what they were told were "the new normal" contours of reality.

Imagine that everyone around you embraced all of the above and undertook public shaming campaigns against anyone who disagreed. Their faces would turn red, and they would shriek in righteous indignation, "Listen to The Science!" whenever anyone attempted to point out the manifest absurdity of what was going on. They would denounce as a degenerate, anti-science, anti-vax ignoramus anyone who pointed out that pharmaceutical firms are profit-driven, publicly traded companies whose success depends on their ability to develop, produce, and market new wares.

7. A Perfect Totalitarian Storm

March 4, 2021
Holladay, Utah

People often express consternation over how something as awful as the Holocaust could ever have transpired. It seems utterly incomprehensible, until one reflects upon the acquiescence to government authorities of individuals, most of whom served as unwitting cogs in a murderous machine. The vast majority of people in 1930s and 1940s Germany went about their business, agreeing to do what officials and bureaucrats told them to do, and brushing aside any questions which may have popped up in their minds about policies preventing Jewish people from holding positions in society and stripping them of their property. For ready identification, Jews were preposterously made to stitch yellow stars onto their clothing. Later, in the concentration camps, they were tattooed with identification numbers. The rest is the grisliest episode in human history.

It is easy to say today, looking back, that we would never have supported the Third Reich and its outrageous laws, but citizens everywhere develop habits of submission to authority from an early age. Many "rule-governed" persons never pause to ask whether the current laws of the land are in fact moral, despite the long history of legislation modified or overturned in the eventual recognition that it was deeply flawed. It is understandable that people should obey the law: they are threatened with punishments, often severe, for failure to comply. But the little things do eventually add up, and one thing leads to another, with the result that the bureaucratic banality of evil diagnosed by Hannah Arendt in her coverage of the Adolf Eichmann trial in 1960 applies every bit as much to our present times as it did to the people going along to get along with the Third Reich.[41] Of course no one is currently sending trainloads of "undesirables" to concentration camps for liquidation, but when one considers the death and degradation of millions of people in the Middle East over the course of the twenty-first century — carnage and misery funded by U.S. taxpayers — one begins to comprehend how the very mentality which permitted the Holocaust to transpire is indeed at work today. The vast majority of Western citizens freely agree to pay their governments to terrorize and attack, even torture, people inhabiting lands far away. The perpetrators call all that they do "national defense," but from the perspective of the victims, the effects are one and the same.

The banality of evil at work today involves a profound complacency among the general populace toward foreign policy. President Biden bombed Syria about a month after becoming the commander-in-chief of the U.S. military, without even seeking congressional authority, and people barely blinked. The elimination of the persons responsible for the terrorist attacks of September 11, 2001, was achieved long ago. Yet military intervention continues on inexorably, having come to be regarded as the rule rather than the exception. The "collateral damage" victims are essentially fictionalized in the minds of the citizens who pay for all of the harm done to them. Habits of deference to the Pentagon and its associated pundits on matters of foreign policy have as their inevitable consequence that confirmed war criminals are permitted to perpetrate their homicidal programs unabated, provided only that they claim to be defending the country, and no matter how disastrous their initiatives proved to be in the past. Indeed, it is difficult to resist the conclusion that the more mistakes a government official makes, the more likely it becomes that he or she will be invited back to serve again, and the more frequently his or her opinion will be sought out by mainstream media outlets.

It requires a type of arrogance to reject the proclamations of the anointed "experts," and in the age of social media, there are always thousands of shills, both paid and unpaid, standing by to defend the programs of the powerful. Antiwar activists are very familiar with how all of this works. They are denounced as unpatriotic, ignorant, naïve, and even evil for refusing to promote the company line. During the Cold War, the reigning false dichotomies of "Capitalist or Communist" and "Patriot or Traitor" held sway, and, sad to say, such false dichotomies abound today. The fact that the pundits and policymakers calling for and applauding military intervention often stand to profit from the campaigns they promote is brushed aside as somehow irrelevant. In contrast, antiwar voices are muted, suppressed, and censored, despite the fact that reasons for opposing more war cannot be said to be tainted by mercenary motives, because peace, unlike war, does not pay.

It costs nothing to *not* bomb a country, so those who speak out against the idea are not doing so in order to profit. Yet such persons are denounced and marginalized in the harshest of terms as cranks, crackpots, extremists, Russia sympathizers, and more. President Obama's drone killing czar John

Brennan famously organized "Terror Tuesday" meetings at the White House, where "suspicious" persons were selected for execution by unmanned combat aerial vehicles (UCAV), a.k.a. lethal drones, on the basis of flash-card presentations crafted from bribed intelligence, drone video footage, and cellphone SIM card data — all of which is circumstantial evidence of the potential for future possible crimes. Brennan recently included libertarians among what he warned is an "unholy alliance" of "domestic extremists" in the wake of the January 6, 2021, protest at the U.S. Capitol.[42] What happens next?

One certainly hopes that educated people are aware that Brennan's inclusion of libertarians among his list of potentially dangerous domestic enemies betrays his utter ignorance of the very meaning of the word *libertarian.* The Non-Aggression Principle (NAP) embraced by libertarians precludes not only wars of aggression but also individual acts of terrorism. Sadly, it has become abundantly clear that the people still watching television news continue to accept and parrot freely what the mass media networks pump out, despite their clearly propagandistic bias in recent years. Accustomed to heeding the prescriptions of "the experts," people blithely listen to Brennan (and those of his ilk) despite his manifest record of duplicity regarding the drone killing campaigns, and his histrionic, even hysterical, comportment during the three-year Russiagate hunt for a Putin-Trump connection.

Neoliberal and neoconservative powerbrokers naturally wish to quash alternative viewpoints, so perhaps no one should be surprised that Brennan has attempted to discredit libertarians. After all, they pose incisive, often disturbing questions, such as whether all of the mass homicide carried out in the name of the nation actually helps anyone, including those paying for the carnage, or rather harms everyone, with the notable exception of those who stand to profit financially or politically from the wars. What Brennan revealed by lumping libertarians together with "domestic terrorists" is that he is not concerned so much with violent threats to the nation but rather with *dissent* from the political and warmaking authorities, a tendency which is becoming more and more marked as the Democratic-controlled Congress attempts to force Big Tech companies such as Facebook and Twitter to "do more" to prevent the dissemination of so-called disinformation. By denouncing some of the most articulate, consistent, and persistent opponents to the war machine as "dangerous," Brennan made it more difficult than it already was for those voices to be heard, much less heeded.

The current complacency of citizens toward U.S. foreign policy is nothing new. Contemporaneously, people anywhere and everywhere tend to go along to get along, whether or not they are convinced that the policies imposed upon them and their fellow citizens make any sense. In 1930s Germany, antisemitism was real, but part of the reason for the efficacy of the nationalist fervor drummed up by Adolf Hitler and used to support his quest for total global domination was the dire economic situation following the loss of World War I. Germany was weak, and its people hungry. Those conditions made it easier than usual to persuade people to comply, in the hope that their lives would be improved by banding together against what was denounced at the time as the evil enemy.

This perennial Manichean trope of political propaganda has most recently emerged in the abject, overt hatred by about half of the people of the United States of anyone having anything whatsoever to do with Donald Trump. "Trump Derangement Syndrome," or TDS, is a genuine phenomenon, at least judging by the comportment of people online and sometimes in person as well. As bizarre as this may be, people actually appear to *hate* people who *do not hate* Donald Trump, having failed to understand that contradictions and contraries are not one and the same. It is entirely possible not to hate Trump while also not loving him, but attempting to elucidate this false dichotomy to anyone who spent the last four years wishing fervently for the former president's demise will be met with an even more strident repetition of the very dichotomy being debunked.

Again, if you happen to believe that the post-presidential impeachment trial was a waste of time and taxpayer money, then you must, according to the anti-Trump mob, love the former president. What is worse, somehow over the course of the past four years a large swath of people have come to believe that seething hatred is a moral virtue, so long as it is directed at appropriate objects of loathing. But the capacity to hate one's fellow human beings reveals absolutely nothing about the hater beyond his ability to hate. It certainly does not mean that he is good by contrast, and it is no mean feat of self-deception to come to believe that because one hates Donald Trump, this alone suffices to establish one's moral superiority over all of the people who do not.

Once people become convinced of their own moral righteousness in the battle against whoever has been designated the evil and benighted (deplorable!) enemy, then it's only a few short steps from "The end justifies the means" to "Everything is permitted." A glaring example has been the more and more prevalent suppression and erasure of so-called disinformation, which of course lies in the eyes of the censors. The necessity of defeating "the enemy" became the basis for such curious developments as the refusal of any of the mass media networks to investigate the pay-for-play connections suggested by the contents of the Hunter Biden laptop made public during the 2020 presidential election cycle. Immediately following Election Day, when some people pointed out anomalies such as the appearance of vertical lines in the graphs of vote tallies in the middle of the night in multiple states — indicating the sudden addition of troves of votes none of which were for Trump — the mass media immediately, in concert, issued headlines everywhere proclaiming that any and all charges of electoral fraud were "baseless." The point here is not that the charges were not baseless, which perhaps they were in some cases — those explained away by local election authorities as clerical errors. But no one could *know* that allegations of electoral fraud were baseless before the matters were investigated.

The slippery slope of censorship is difficult to resist, having taken the first step onto that totalitarian-veering path, and the removal from social media of thousands of conservative and right-wing accounts regarded as sympathetic with Trump and his gallery of rogues is simply not enough, according to Democratic Party elites. Despite having already propagandized much of the mainstream media (as was evident in the election and post-election coverage), the Democrats, giddy with their majority Blue-Blue-Blue capture of Washington, now wish to exert total control over what people may say, write, and read. This is, of course, a violation of the First Amendment of the Constitution of the United States, but by achieving their goal through the indirect manipulation of private companies, which are subject to federal regulation and therefore receptive to "innuendos" on the part of legislators, they are hoping that no one will notice what has transpired — at least not before it is too late to do anything about it.

After Trump's acquittal in the second Senate impeachment trial, the news coverage claiming that he had incited "insurrection" at the Capitol continued on, as though the facts had already been established and the outcome of the trial was entirely irrelevant. These Associated Press (AP) excerpts are typical:

> "The only president to be impeached twice has once again evaded consequences..." (February 13, 2021)
>
> "After [Trump] incited a deadly riot at the U.S. Capitol last month..." (February 14, 2021)

One might with reason wonder whether the wrongness of questioning the outcome of an election does not imply the wrongness of questioning the outcome of a trial. Of course, both are perfectly permissible in a society which champions freedom of speech. What this political control of the news reveals is a republic in crisis, for if even supposedly objective news outlets such as the Associated Press reject the outcome of processes intended to ascertain the truth, then the people have no way of being able to determine what actually transpired. Similar examples of journalistic *léger-de-main* abound in every area of importance to neoliberals — above all, in matters of war — and the mainstream media's refusal even to discuss the plight of Julian Assange is a case in point. Assange made public evidence of war crimes committed by the U.S. government but is now being persecuted as though *he* were a murderer. So pathological has the mainstream press become that the only times they were able to bring themselves to praise Trump was when he ordered military strikes on the people of the Middle East.

The tech outlets have now also decided to censor alleged disinformation about the experimental mRNA COVID-19 vaccines, conflating the criticisms of persons opposed to all vaccines (the anti-vaxxers) with those of persons who have read the spec sheets, are aware of the data on disease prognosis, and find that the risk of possible, as-of-yet unknown long-term side effects are not outweighed by the alleged benefits of the novel technology (which, it is worth pointing out, never made it past the animal trials when it was tested in the past). Those who express concern about the Procrustean lockdowns have also been subjected to suppression of their speech. The Facebook page for the Great Barrington Declaration[43] was taken down by censors, and Robert F. Kennedy, Jr.'s Children's Health Defense[44] organization has also been deplatformed. But the criticisms offered by these groups are grounded in scientific literature. Indeed, the authors of the Great Barrington Declaration are in fact epidemiologists and public health scientists, but they are summarily dismissed as quacks because they disagree with the Fauci-Gates program.

What the vast majority of people want is for the current abnormal situation to be stabilized. If that means embracing what the powers that be are calling "the new normal," then so be it. Anyone who stands in the way of the needed changes — those who refuse to volunteer as unpaid subjects in the largest experimental trial of a novel medical device in history — are summarily denounced in the usual terms: selfish, deplorable, ignorant, inbred, racist, nutjobs, etc. It does not matter in the least whether any of the epithets are true. They are deployed indiscriminately against anyone who disagrees by the self-styled morally superior types who shill for the reigning political and corporate elites — often for free.

The present circumstances offer the necessary prerequisites to totalitarianism. We would do well to heed the historical record and look closely at how Nazism and Stalinism became dominant outlooks for entire populations, despite the fact that large numbers of people were destroyed by them. The total control of the mainstream media, with a specific agenda being promoted, all alternatives suppressed, and the extreme polarization of citizens under Manichean false dichotomies, is everywhere on display. What's more, in these COVIDystopic times, we are witnessing people struggling under the same economic hardships as were the people of 1930s Germany. What is worse, after a full year of non-stop television coverage of death tolls, with nearly no effort by any mainstream pundits to place the tallies into proper context and consider how many people were dying every day before COVID-19 arrived on the scene, many citizens are understandably afraid.

Fear always brings out the worst in groups of people, who may team up against what they decry as the evil enemy. But fear, hatred, and self-deception conjoined produce a toxic soup, and we need not search the annals of the first half of the twentieth century to find evidence of this. Post-9/11, violent crimes against Muslim people (and other brown-skinned persons sometimes mistaken for "Arabs") were on the rise. We are currently on a trajectory leading to a place where those who read the spec sheets for the "free" vaccines and then, based on that information, decline to roll up their sleeves, will be denigrated as criminals. The divisions being concretized between those healthy, robust people who agree to COVID-19 vaccination and those who demur are being strengthened by virtue-signaling campaigns making everyone who gets the vaccine believe, again, amazingly enough, that they are morally superior to those who do not. Even Britain's Queen Elizabeth has come out to denounce publicly those who have declined to participate in the experimental vaccine trials as "selfish."[45]

Technocrats the world over have been warning since at least April 2020 that the only way out of our current predicament will be to issue "vaccine passports" through which the healthy can be distinguished from the unhealthy. However, even if the first and second round of vaccines together work to prevent transmission and infection — which has yet to be established — those who have received them will not be protected from the new variants, and will need to submit to a third round of so-called booster shots, which in another six months will likely "require" a fourth booster, and so on. All of this would seem to imply that the "vaccine passports" being floated by government and corporate leaders will in no way ensure that the persons carrying them are not going to contract or transmit the latest variants of the virus. So what do they really mean?

The idea that those who have accepted COVID-19 vaccines are "fit to fly," to work, to socialize, or even to go outside, rests on a truly Orwellian redefinition of "healthy" as "vaccinated," even as scientists continue to warn that the virus has already transformed enough to check the already questionable efficacy of the current crop of vaccines. Those who support the implementation of vaccine passports are fond of pointing out that people traveling to Africa are required first to be vaccinated against Yellow Fever. But COVID-19 is nothing like Yellow Fever, which kills half of the people it infects. The vast majority of persons do not need to introduce foreign substances into their body in order to survive COVID-19. Because the vaccines appear to mitigate serious symptoms and increase the odds of survival among vulnerable persons, they should of course be offered the option of vaccination, but it must remain their choice, for they alone will bear the brunt of any untoward side effects, which invariably arise in a small portion of the population with every vaccine.

In the Nuremberg trials, nonconsensual human experimentation was decried and judged to be a crime against humanity (see Appendix B). But extortion, too, is a form of coercion, and we should not be fooled by the latest Newspeak press releases in which "authorities" attempt both to cajole and to threaten us for defying their will. Former U.K. Prime Minister (and confirmed war criminal[46]) Tony Blair has determined that vaccine passports will be our ticket to freedom.[47] This is a shocking pronouncement because our freedom is not his or anyone else's to withhold from us, least of all when our own persons and bodies are at stake. It's as though we are currently inhabiting an episode of *Black Mirror*, where the dark heart of pharma-technocratic rule is working to bend us to its will, using compliant *citoyens* as its unwitting tools. Peer pressure, shaming, bribes, and threats are nothing new, but in this case the consequences could not be more personal.

History clearly demonstrates that one repressive measure leads to another, and totalitarianism creeps in step by step, unnoticed until it is too late. From the suppression of speech, to the lockdown and quarantine of healthy people, to coercing or extorting them to participate in experimental trials — none of this bodes well for the future of freedom. The fight to retain what are our rights — to speech, liberty, privacy, and the pursuit of happiness — and above all not to be treated as the possessions of government-funded corporations, must be defended while this is still possible. When a system is sufficiently infiltrated at every stratum by fanatics convinced of their own moral superiority and monopoly on the truth, then totalitarianism is near. It happened in Nazi Germany, and it happened in Stalin's Soviet Union. We are moving perilously close to that nightmarish reality right here and now, as people redefine basic terms such as *sickness* and *health* and insist on exerting total control over information flow.

8. Pascal's Wager for COVIDystopic Times, or: How I Learned to Stop Worrying About the Coronapocalypse and Eat Krispy Kreme Doughnuts

April 2, 2021
Holladay, Utah

Being of a naturally skeptical bent, I have harbored doubts from the very beginning about the upheaval of the entire world rationalized by politicians everywhere because of a virus which kills less than 1% of the people it infects. I watched in amazement as country after country closed their borders to foreigners, imposed "common sense" quarantines, lockdowns, and mask mandates, and shut down entire economies. I was perplexed by the inability of anyone in the position to craft policies to recognize that what really needed to be done was to isolate vulnerable persons, allow everyone else to go about their business, and eventually we would achieve herd immunity.

This approach was rejected early on as untenable because, it was claimed, COVID-19 was simply too elusive. In contrast to many other deadly viruses known to mankind since time immemorial, we could not develop herd immunity to COVID-19, because there were documented cases of persons who had become reinfected after having already recovered. To my mind, that was a red flag that perhaps the virus had not simply leapt from bats to humans when some hapless soul in Wuhan ate a bowl of soup. I wondered whether this was not some sort of Frankenstein gain-of-function virus, engineered in a lab by DARPA-funded scientists under the guise of national defense, to figure out what to do in case some other government developed such a virus to wipe out its sworn enemies.

The idea that COVID-19 was developed in a lab and released by human error was rejected by all of the CNN-certified authorities, so I naturally listened to "The Science" and began focusing on other matters, such as whether the project of inoculating all of the 9 billion people on the planet with a vaccine might be a way of ending the pandemic. There were plenty of companies enthusiastic to pursue this project, and within months Pfizer, Moderna, AstraZeneca, and Johnson & Johnson, in addition to a variety of companies in Russia and China, had already developed their vaccines, having been generously funded by governments so obviously keen to save lives.

Fine, I thought to myself. Now everyone who is vulnerable can get the vaccine, and those who are not can go about their business, become infected, and then recover from the virus and its associated symptoms upon robust people, such as the "blah" feeling reported by Tom Hanks upon landing on Australian shores in March 2020 shortly before that entire country closed its borders seemingly forever.[48] There was no question in my mind that we were on the way to the exit ramp of the highway to a dystopic world where no one is allowed to travel or congregate in groups for fear of transmitting the virus to persons who might die as a result. The situation was easy to comprehend by appeal to Pascal's wager (*mutatis mutandis*):

The Question of Efficacy in Preventing Transmission and Infection

	Take the Vaccine	Don't Take the Vaccine
The vaccine prevents transmission and infection.	Everyone who takes the vaccine will be protected from everyone else — whether or not they take the vaccine.	Those who take the vaccine will be protected; others will remain vulnerable to COVID-19.
The vaccine does not prevent transmission and infection.	No one who takes the vaccine will be protected from other people — whether or not they take the vaccine.	No one will be protected — whether or not they take the vaccine.

Further doubts, however, began to creep into my mind as I witnessed a variety of zealous public relations efforts to persuade people invulnerable to COVID-19 to get the vaccines. Front and center in luring the public to do what the CDC has determined must be done are COVID-19 guru Dr. Anthony Fauci and vaccine entrepreneur Bill Gates, who incidentally has revealed in interviews his fabulous financial success in the vaccine sector. I think that everyone, on both sides of the COVID-19 lockdown divide, can agree that a twentyfold return on his investment is nothing to scoff at.[49]

Fauci got right to work promoting the Moderna vaccine by pointing out to African Americans that, in fact, the vaccine was developed by a black woman. This struck me as an odd selling point, and I confess to have suspected racism. I looked up Dr. Kizzmekia Corbett on Twitter and found this on her profile: "Virology. Vaccinology. Vagina-ology. Vino-ology." Not sure that the latter two count as credentials, but one thing is clear: vaccine hesitancy among African Americans has a well-documented and understandable history, resulting in part from the horrifying Tuskegee experiments, in which black men infected with syphilis were left untreated "just to see what would happen." That's right: nonconsensual human experimentation was not the province only of the Nazis. It has happened right here in the United States as well.

In turning Dr. Corbett into something of a media darling, Fauci's idea appears to have been that people would be persuaded that a black woman would never dream of acting so as to harm other black people. That line of argumentation is unfortunately impugned by the fact that black nurses were among the perpetrators of the Tuskegee study.[50] Indeed, the program coordinator, Eunice Verdell Rivers Laurie,[51] was an African American woman. Nonetheless, Fauci may have succeeded in convincing some people to roll up their sleeves, to wit, those entirely ignorant of the details of the disturbing Tuskegee saga, which lasted a shocking forty years.

My next concern arose when some "experts" began exhorting pregnant women to "get the jab," insisting that there was no evidence of harm to pregnant women from the new vaccines. I decided to look into the studies done before the emergency authorizations and discovered that pregnant women were not included in the first round of human trials. This finding naturally reminded me of the horror story of Thalidomide.[52] That drug seemed very safe in initial clinical trials, which, however, excluded pregnant women. Ultimately, 40% of the babies of women who had been given Thalidomide as a remedy for morning sickness died around the time of birth. Of those who survived, thousands were born deformed, many with fin-like limbs. As is always the case, it took time for the long-term side effects to be sorted out. That is because each patient is unique, with different biological and environmental factors, including the medical treatment in question, acting upon her body. Approved in 1956, Thalidomide was not pulled from the European market until 1961.

Why would anyone be encouraging pregnant women to "get the jab," given the well-documented history of Thalidomide and the apparent invulnerability of infants and small children to the COVID-19 virus? I puzzled. After all, the word *teratogen* exists because there are substances which predictably lead to birth defects, and they are discovered when, and only when, pregnant women are exposed to those substances. Thinking about the case of Thalidomide and possible side effects provoked another Pascal's Wager assessment:

The Question of Unknown Side Effects — Both Short-Term and Long-Term

	Take the Vaccine	**Don't Take the Vaccine**
The vaccine prevents transmission and infection.	Those who take the vaccine will be protected from COVID-19 but may suffer side effects — up to and including death.	Those who do not take the vaccine will not be protected from COVID-19 but will not suffer any side effects.
The vaccine does not prevent transmission and infection.	Those who take the vaccine will not be protected from COVID-19 and may also suffer side effects — up to and including death.	Those who do not take the vaccine will not be protected from COVID-19 but will also not suffer any side effects.

The worst-case scenario would be that the "vaccines" do not actually work and also have devastating side effects. Clearly, then, the rational choice for a given person is going to be a function of how vulnerable he or she is to the disease which the vaccines are intended to protect against. If one has a greater than 99.5% chance of surviving COVID-19, has no known comorbidities, and therefore is unlikely to suffer severe illness, even if infected with the virus, then it is difficult to see why he or she would want to opt for the treatment, given that the risk of long-term side effects is *entirely unknown* — ranging anywhere from 0% to 100%. *Fine*, I concluded again. People who want the vaccine can get the vaccine, and everyone else can resume normal life. Yet Fauci & Co. did not agree. I continued to puzzle over pregnant women being enthusiastically exhorted to "get the jab," and those concerns were exacerbated when vaccine trials on children began, complete with a social media campaign featuring images of "heroic" pro-science kids rolling up their sleeves.

Eventually, after reflecting on this conundrum for quite some time, the firm believer in freedom of choice in me capitulated, concluding that, as in everything else, parents and pregnant women would have to decide what to do for themselves and their offspring. I decided to move on to other matters, as it was obviously futile to engage further with the mobs of people online who have redefined "prudential person" to mean "anti-vaxxer." Instead, I turned to the rational grounds for believing that Moderna and its diverse research team have succeeded in producing a COVID-19 *vaccine*, which used to be defined by the CDC as follows:

> *vaccine*: a product that stimulates a person's immune system to produce immunity to a specific disease, protecting the person from that disease.[53]

Going directly to the source, Moderna's own website,[54] I learned that the company specializes in gene therapy and has been operational for a grand total of ten years. They received a substantial DARPA grant in 2013 but have no FDA approvals for vaccines or devices to date, aside from the Emergency Use Authorization (EUA) granted in December 2020 for the COVID-19 treatment. All of the COVID-19 therapies, whether mRNA (as in Moderna's case) or vector-based, have been labeled "vaccines" not only in the hope that they *may* act as vaccines, but also in order to benefit from the legal immunity enjoyed by vaccine manufacturers in the United States, thanks to the PREP (Public Readiness and Emergency Preparedness) Act.[55] Anyone who suffers harm as a result of these government-funded elixirs will have to take it up with the government, not the manufacturer.

Unlike normal businesses, which must bear the legal brunt of the negative effects of their products upon human beings, Moderna is like a child being allowed to roam free, its parents prepared to clean up any messes which may result. Perhaps Moderna will get lucky and have produced a miracle cure, but the statistics on new medical treatments are not that encouraging. Of 5,000 new drug candidates, only a tiny fraction of them (5 out of 5,000, or 0.1%) are judged from the animal trials to be safe enough to be tested on human beings.[56] Of those which are tested on human beings, only 20% eventually achieve (regular) FDA approval and are taken to market (0.02% of the original candidates). Of those pharmaceutical products which make it to market, some are eventually recalled. From January 2017 to September 2019, 195 drugs previously approved by the FDA were recalled because of safety issues.[57]

Now, many people have died of COVID-19, and no one wishes for that to happen to himself or anyone he knows. It is also true that very ill and vulnerable people are often willing to gamble on experimental treatments. In the case of terminally ill patients, what do they have to lose? It is unclear, however, why any rational person not at risk of death from COVID-19 should want to offer up, without compensation, his healthy body as a Petri dish to a government-subsidized and protected industry with a well-documented history of not only deception and fraud but also what are arguably human rights violations, above all, in Third World countries. Moderna, being new, with no products on the market, has a clean slate to date (all *none* of its products have had no untoward effects on human subjects), but the Pfizer, Johnson & Johnson, and AstraZeneca tallies of criminal fines and settlements are awe-inspiring, to put it mildly.[58] No one ever said that human experimentation was going to be risk-free, but the fact that billions of dollars in compensations have been doled out to people harmed by pharmaceutical and other chemical companies underscores a sober truth: it is inherently dangerous to introduce novel foreign substances into human bodies, even in the best of all possible research and development scenarios.

The spec sheets for both the Pfizer[59] and the Moderna[60] shots explicitly state that they "may" prevent one from getting COVID-19 (which implies, of course, that they may not) and that "there is no FDA-approved vaccine to prevent COVID-19." These information sheets (which hardly any people rolling up their sleeves appear to have read) also state plainly that "serious and unexpected side effects may occur," which should in any case be obvious since they were developed and tested over a course of months, not years. (Note: the average time to market for a new drug/device is twelve years.) There simply is no long-term data yet, whether positive or negative. The makers themselves of these products rightly express ignorance as to their efficacy in preventing and transmitting disease, touting confidently only their therapeutic effect in reducing severe symptoms and diminishing the likelihood of death, both of which are in any case exceedingly rare for persons under the age of fifty, according to all available statistical data. Feeling "blah" does not count, I presume, as a "severe symptom," so it is unclear whether vaccination would have helped Tom Hanks at all. *But who knows? One or more of these companies may succeed in producing a COVID-19 panacea,* I mused. Until I remembered the problem of new virus variants.

The current slate of vaccines were developed against a dominant strain of COVID-19 last year, but the many variants, created through mutation and apparently numbering in the thousands, are by now so widespread that there are grounds for believing that even if the current vaccines work against the dominant strain, and even with strong vaccine compliance, vulnerable people will continue to die, sooner or later, while everyone else will be spared, not because of the vaccines, but because they were never vulnerable to the virus and its variants in the first place. As is always the case, given human variability, there have been some outliers, young persons who died or suffered harm from SARS-CoV-2 infection. On the other hand, more elderly people than one might surmise, given the media coverage, have survived. COVID-19 does not come close to being a death sentence, although the chances of dying are significantly increased for patients with comorbidities. Still, in some places, the average age of a COVID-19 victim is the same or even older than the average life expectancy of people more generally.[61]

Curiously enough, persons who already survived COVID-19 are also being exhorted to get the vaccines, even though the very fact of their ongoing existence definitively demonstrates that their immune system is hardy enough to combat the virus. For other diseases caused by viruses and for which vaccines exist, the reason for getting the vaccine is to avoid at all costs getting the disease, which in cases such as Ebola and Yellow Fever are very deadly to anyone, regardless of age or comorbidities. But the vast majority of people infected with COVID-19 experience only mild symptoms and do not require medical treatment. Reflecting on these matters, I circled back to my previous concern: *Why should any healthy person believe that taking an experimental vaccine is a good idea, particularly if he or she already survived COVID-19?*

As I continued to mull over this question, I marveled at the massive media marketing budget for COVID-19. All the circular stickers on the ground and all the signs everywhere relaying important information such as the permitted capacity of persons inside stores, all scientifically calculated to three significant figures to yield numbers such as the 163 shoppers admitted to the local TJ Maxx at a time. Even more impressive have been the ads on television and the Internet everywhere encouraging people: "This is our shot. Let's take it!" among a slate of similarly benevolent-sounding slogans. People may feel better when others hop aboard the vaccine train, and they may attempt to shame those who do not, but does any of this behavior have anything to do with whether or not the treatments will ultimately work? It seems safe to say that neither the virus nor the vaccines have any interest in the hopes and aspirations of human beings. Ironically, the pressure being put on people — threatening the requirement of vaccination for travel, work, and play, and the lavishing of praise upon those willing blindly to accept as-of-yet unknown risks — appears to be having the opposite of its intended effect.

If it were so obvious that the vaccines worked and were the only solution to our current predicament, then why would Queen Elizabeth take to the airwaves to denounce people who refuse to get vaccinated as "selfish"? Why would Tony Blair insist that we will not be free again until vaccine passports become available? Why did former Presidents Bill Clinton, George W. Bush, and Barack Obama team up to produce a video in which they attempt to persuade people to get the vaccine? (Bush states in the ad, "The science is clear." He was equally confident about Saddam Hussein's WMD.) Why would CNN be admonishing[62] those congresspersons who have declined the vaccines made available to them, including Representative Thomas Massie and others who have already recovered from the virus and therefore must have developed antibodies and T-cells in response?[63] On its face, all of this propaganda seems vaguely insane, and it is scaring people away who might otherwise have agreed to participate in the experimental trials.

Sowing doubts even more effectively than appeals by confirmed liars in high places, more than twenty countries, including France, Germany, Italy, Norway, Finland, Thailand, and, most recently, Canada, halted their distribution of the Oxford/AstraZeneca vaccine in response to a number of blood clot cases. When the cases in Norway were first reported, the trusty mainstream media went into overdrive, dismissing "baseless" claims of connections between the blood clots and the vaccine. It seemed strange to me that over the course of the past year, every person who died *with* COVID-19 was recorded as having died *of* COVID-19, while no one who died after vaccination was acknowledged to have been killed by the vaccine. That the (in some cases) deadly blood clots were "purely coincidental" was the judgment decreed by journalists onboard the vaccine train before the matter was even investigated, and echoed by parrots throughout Facebook and Twitter to assuage the fears of persons who might be discouraged by the news from rolling up their sleeves.

Even after the AstraZeneca vaccination programs resumed in most of the countries which had paused their use, some of them changed their guidelines. France, for example, having initially claimed that the AstraZeneca vaccine showed no benefits to elderly persons, reversed course to decree that the vaccine should *only* be used on persons over the age of 55. Canada, for its part, announced that they would be administering the AstraZeneca vaccine only to persons between the ages of 50 and 65. The governments which stopped and then resumed vaccination claimed that they had done so out of "an abundance of caution," but when some scientists concluded that there was indeed a connection between the blood clots and a rare autoimmune response elicited by the vaccine,[64] they also jubilantly reported that they had found a possible cure for that problem. *By all means, take the AstraZeneca vaccine, and if you develop blood clots in your brain, then we'll give you some other treatment to save your life!* (If you have no Big Pharma stocks in your portfolio, now might be the time to buy.)

Many businesses have joined in on the public relations campaign and are rising to the challenge of convincing their customers that vaccination is the way to go. Qantas, the largest Australian airline, has adopted the punitive approach, alerting all passengers everywhere that they will not be boarding any of their planes without first presenting proof of vaccination. But one company has gone above and beyond to offer what may finally be needed to convert the intransigent skeptics: Krispy Kreme. The doughnut giant has announced that anyone presenting proof of vaccination at any of their stores will be entitled to a free doughnut.[65] Mind you, this is not a one-off promotion. All vaccinated persons are being offered a doughnut every single day that they show up at any of the Krispy Kreme locations with a trusty vaccination card in hand. Needless to say, this propitious development necessitates a revision of the Pascal's Wager assessment:

To Vaccinate, or Not to Vaccinate?

	Take the Vaccine	**Don't Take the Vaccine**
The vaccine prevents transmission and infection.	Those who take the vaccine will be protected from COVID-19 and will receive a free doughnut every day.	Those who do not take the vaccine will not be protected from COVID-19 and will not receive a free doughnut every day.
The vaccine does not prevent transmission and infection.	Those who take the vaccine will not be protected from COVID-19 but will receive a free doughnut every day.	Those who do not take the vaccine will not be protected from COVID-19 and will not receive a free doughnut every day.

Luckily, there are Krispy Kreme doughnut shops dotting the vast landscape of the United States, and, more importantly, there is one down the street from me. My fate, therefore, along with that of thousands, if not millions, of my fellow citizens (including, I presume, Representative Massie), is now sealed. I will be rolling up my sleeve, not because I believe in the novel mRNA vaccines, nor because I think that it is in my best interests to undergo an experimental treatment for a disease to which I am not vulnerable and from which I have already recovered, nor because George W. Bush and Tony Blair want me to, nor because I care what Queen Elizabeth thinks of me, nor because the only way I can ever travel to Australia again will be to "get the jab." No, I will be rolling up my sleeve for the sole purpose of receiving a free doughnut every day henceforth. I trust that, in recognition of the Krispy Kreme executive team's manifest magnanimity, the government will confer upon their company the label "essential business" to protect it from revenue loss in the event of any future lockdowns.

9. Moral Rhetoric versus Reality

May 13, 2021
Bothell, Washington

Philosophers tend to divide normative theories of morality into two broad categories: deontological and teleological. Deontological theories prioritize right action over good outcomes. If an action is wrong, then it is intrinsically wrong, regardless of the consequences which may ensue. The Ten Commandments and Kant's Categorical Imperative are classic examples of deontological theories, and the libertarian Non-Aggression Principle (NAP) is another one: *Do not initiate violence against any person, or damage or steal his property.* Teleological theories, in contrast, define *rightness* in terms of *goodness.* One determines what to do in part — if not exclusively — by considering the likely outcomes or consequences of one's prospective action.

Arguably the most famous teleological theory is utilitarianism, articulated by British thinkers Jeremy Bentham and John Stuart Mill in the late eighteenth and early nineteenth centuries. According to the simplest formulation of utilitarianism, what one should do is always act so as to maximize the good outcomes (happiness or pleasure or something else positive — Bentham and Mill called this "utility") and minimize the bad outcomes (unhappiness or pain or something else negative) for the greatest number of people. Without delving too deeply into what consistently applied utilitarianism would actually entail, the idea seems *prima facie* reasonable to many, and it is appealing to "social justice warriors" and others who believe that the government has and should play an important role in improving the lot of the citizenry through engineering the society in which they live. This basic outlook informs socialist economic theories according to which wealth should be redistributed so that the goods of society are shared rather than "hoarded" by the small percentage of the population comprising the elites.

The theoretical problem with utilitarianism is that there is no hard limit on what can be done to a few people in the name of the net good of the greater group. Everything is, in principle, permissible, depending only on the context and likely consequences. If torturing or killing one innocent person will save the rest of humanity, then it may in fact be the right thing to do, according to utilitarianism. The hypothetical scenarios used to elicit utilitarian responses tend to be highly simplistic, such as the "Trolley

Problem" discussed in many college ethics courses. One version of the Trolley Problem involves a conductor who must decide whether to kill five people (say, senior citizens) on one track, or to divert his car to another track and kill three other people (say, toddlers) thereby. Those who devise such thought experiments are attempting to isolate the variables, rendering it possible to gauge sympathies for or against utilitarianism in spite of the inherent complexities of reality.

Because human beings live in societies, the political realm abounds with utilitarian-esque rationalizations for anything and everything. Currently, many of those calling for universal vaccination against COVID-19 are reasoning as utilitarians when they presume that the relatively small number of outlier deaths and severe harm caused to a few of those vaccinated will be vastly outweighed by the lives saved. Those who decline vaccination are denounced in the harshest of terms as "selfish," when in fact they may simply disagree with either the projected result (that millions of people will be saved from the virus and few killed by the vaccines) or else the risk calculation in their own case, based on the statistical data for COVID-19 vulnerability and the complete absence of data on long-term vaccine side effects.

That competent individuals alone should make determinations for themselves of which risks to assume is a deontological position, denying as it does that "the greater good" is a sound pretext for stripping persons of their liberty and right to control their own body. Forced vaccination would constitute a flagrant violation of the libertarian's NAP, so for libertarians who support universal vaccination, the only consistent approach is to *persuade* others to join them in rolling up their sleeves.

On the economic front, one occasionally finds people today explicitly asserting that humanity would be much better off, for example, if all of Amazon founder Jeff Bezos's massive wealth were taken from him and used to put an end to world hunger. The people who make such suggestions (when they are serious) appear to assume that the accumulation of wealth is a zero-sum game, and they reject the "trickle-down" economic theories which may inform a more liberty-forward approach.[66] Supporters of a socialist agenda are wont to ignore the lessons of failed experiments such as that of the former Soviet Union, maintaining that, if only socialism were implemented correctly, then the world would be a better place. Needless to say, the persons to be harmed in such hypothetical scenarios tend not to agree with what would be the sacrifice of themselves or their property for the greater good of everyone else. Senators Bernie Sanders and Elizabeth Warren, for example, have been known to take aim at Bezos despite the fact that both of these senators own multiple houses but neither offers them (as far as I know) as shelter to persons worse off than themselves. Critiques of the "failure" of Amazon to pay any taxes are especially odd coming from the very legislators who write and ratify laws which permit companies to take advantage of loopholes in order to avoid paying taxes.

In any case, the same critique, that our society tolerates "obscene" disparities in wealth, can be directed toward anyone whose material conditions are significantly better than anyone else's — which is arguably everyone in the United States, all of whom are better off than most of the people inhabiting Third World countries — and yet chooses not to redistribute his own property. As much as caricatures may abound of libertarians as rich, old, white men unwilling to share their wealth with the descendants of the victims whom their great-great-grandparents oppressed, no one agitating for the mass redistribution of other people's wealth need be taken seriously unless he makes himself into the extraordinarily rare example of someone willing to invite everyone less well-off than himself into his own home. Until their comportment is modified to match their rhetoric, the shrill virtue-signaling of Bezos haters and others of their ilk can be safely ignored.

Needless to say, such conflicts between moral rhetoric and reality are ubiquitous. People who denounce manmade climate change sometimes fly to global warming conferences in private jets. Nor do those who incessantly warn about global warming typically renounce their private cars, even when they live in cities with efficient public transportation systems. People who express concern about environmental pollution and the ocean life blighted by plastic waste may nonetheless continue to imbibe water from single-use bottles. That moral rhetoric and reality so often diverge illustrates the practical problem with implementing anything even vaguely approaching utilitarianism, and is metaphorically expressed by George Orwell's *Animal Farm.* The truth is that human beings, as a matter of fact, care much more about themselves and their family members and friends than random compatriots. Moreover, they largely ignore the plight of persons beyond their own borders, even when the taxes levied on their personal income have been used to generate widespread misery abroad. It is utilitarian-esque reasoning when someone claims that wars may harm some people but on balance serve the aims of democracy and peace. Most of the victims of wars over the past century have been unarmed civilians, not soldiers, but their "sacrifice" is nonetheless reimagined by those who support every new war proposed as having contributed to the establishment of a better world.

The prevalence of this type of rhetoric, and its associated pseudo-moral rationalizations for policies which harm or even destroy other people, explains bizarre phenomena such as Speaker of the House of Representatives Nancy Pelosi's public expression of gratitude to George Floyd for having been killed by police officer Derek Chauvin.[67] She spoke directly to the dead man, specifically thanking him for "sacrificing your life for justice." Many people found Pelosi's statement inappropriate and tone-deaf, but she was essentially reciting a version of the same script which is rehearsed every single time soldiers are sacrificed needlessly and so-called "collateral damage" is "tolerated" in wars perpetrated abroad. Slogans such as "Freedom is not free!" are frequently slung about by military supporters, who assume that, on balance, the comportment of the U.S. Department of Defense has been good, even if mistakes are sometimes made, and even if a few "bad apples" emerge here and there to perpetrate the occasional atrocity, for example at My Lai or in the Abu Ghraib and Bagram prisons. Judging by their docile acceptance of the foreign policy of Bush, Obama, Trump, and now Biden, most Americans have yet to acknowledge that the twenty-year "Global War on Terror" (GWOT) was a colossal failure: politically, economically, and, yes, morally. The only people to have benefited from the non-stop bombing of the Middle East are war profiteers. *Some people are more equal than others.*

The long-entrenched dogma that, all things considered, the world is a better place because of U.S. military intervention abroad explains why citizens continue dutifully to pay federal taxes while delegating all policymaking decisions to the legislature, who in the twenty-first century flatly renounced their authority to decide when and where war should be waged. The AUMF (Authorization for Use of Military Force) granted to President George W. Bush in October 2002 has been invoked by every president since then to claim the authority to bomb anyone anywhere in the world where the executive branch of government has deemed such action desirable.

"We are good, and they are evil" is a time-tested trope which allows government administrators, whether elected or appointed by those elected, to get away with anything, on the pretext that the evil enemy must be defeated, and the perpetrators of mass homicide are acting only and everywhere so as to protect their constituents. Or to spread democracy and save the world from a despicable tyrant, all of which are essentially equivalent — or so the rhetoric goes… In the lead-up to every new war, citizens, having been subjected to vigorous fearmongering propaganda campaigns according to which their very lives are at stake, tend to forget momentarily that politicians are liars. They listen attentively as quasi-utilitarianism is trotted out yet again to secure popular support for bombing campaigns through soundbites such as: "The war will pay for itself!" "We will be welcomed with flowers as liberators!" "The conflict will be short — in and out — with minimal collateral damage!" When the real consequences prove to be nothing like those projected by hawkish "experts" with financial ties to military industry, the warmakers then revert to defending themselves by appeal to their good intentions.

War advocates are able to sleep at night not because of utilitarianism, according to which the rightness of a war is determined by its outcomes, which any rational and informed person must own have been catastrophic throughout the Middle East, but because they have another theory to whip out in their defense whenever their "good wars" have infelicitous or even appalling consequences. That framework derives from just war theory, specifically, the doctrine of double effect, according to which what *really* matter, in the grand scheme of things, are the warmakers' own intentions.[68]

"Stuff happens," explained former Secretary of Defense and sage epistemologist Donald Rumsfeld in assuaging concerns that the conditions on the ground in Iraq were chaotic, with monuments and museums being looted, and persons murdered, maimed, robbed, and raped, among other unanticipated results of the 2003 bombing campaign.

Policymakers such as George W. Bush, Dick Cheney, Condoleezza Rice, Paul Wolfowitz, and Tony Blair may assuage their conscience by professing the purity of their own, subjective, intentions: "We meant to do well!" Along these lines, ancient Greek philosopher Socrates reputedly quipped, "No one knowingly does evil," by which he may have meant that everyone seeks what he regards as good and avoids what he regards as evil. What, after all, could we base our actions on, if not our own values? In other words, viewed at the level of individual action, "We meant to do well!" may hold true in the case of anyone who does anything, from the thief who steals to feed his family, to the serial killer who derives immense pleasure from destroying other people, to the war hawks and profiteers who persist in perpetuating and even expanding the "War on Terror," even though it has already destroyed or degraded the lives of thousands of Americans and millions of persons of color abroad.

Some people are more equal than others is assumed by anyone who claims to wish to even the economic playing field at home while altogether ignoring the plight of the millions of people who are not only not earning $15 per hour for their labor but in fact have been *killed* as the so-called "collateral damage" of wars supported or condoned by lawmakers with financial interests at stake. The forever war in the Middle East and Africa plods on with little protest, and some of the very people who vociferously demand justice for individual victims of police brutality such as George Floyd turn a blind eye to the plight of the thousands of victims of the bombing campaigns, despite the fact that the former can be said to derive in part from the latter. Not only does the federal government set a highly visible example of how to resolve conflict through the continual perpetration of mass homicide, but police departments have been furnished with military equipment and are staffed in many places by veterans of U.S. wars, some of whom apply wartime techniques and tactics in combating crime.

With regard to the killing of persons of color within the United States, we have witnessed former President Barack Obama making public pronouncements on the outcomes of the George Floyd and Trayvon Martin cases, while declining to say anything whatsoever about his very own administration's targeted killing of sixteen-year-old Abdulrahman al-Awlaki, a U.S. citizen incinerated along with a group of his friends by a missile launched by the U.S. government from a drone flying above Yemen in 2011.[69] If presidents themselves can simply pretend that some of their very own victims never even existed, then it should not be all that surprising when Americans more generally follow their lead.

Self-styled progressives, for example, may agitate for the restriction of firearm possession domestically, while ignoring altogether the exportation of weapons in record numbers (since Obama's presidency) to regimes and factions in Syria and other places where they are predictably used to harm human beings, primarily persons of color, on a completely different magnitude than occurs within the country where the weapons are produced. It is of course possible to maintain consistently, as do advocates of the right to bear arms, that guns are morally neutral but become implements of murder when wielded by murderers. But anyone who insists that gun possession leads to murder within the United States would seem to be committed, logically speaking, to the position that the many innocent persons killed abroad by U.S. weapons — whether by the U.S. military itself or by governments, factions, or individuals armed by them — were, materially speaking, the murder victims of those who furnished the killers with the weapons. And yet some (not all) of those who dispute citizens' Constitutional right to bear arms are not only silent on the issue of weapons exportation but in fact complicit in enriching this industry and sowing the seeds for mass homicide abroad through their uninterrupted payment of federal taxes.

A similarly untenable duality would seem to be Senator Bernie Sanders's outspoken opposition to capital punishment, which he manages to hold within his mind while simultaneously supporting the use of unmanned combat aerial vehicles (UCAVs), or lethal drones, to kill terrorist suspects abroad. One of the most cogent arguments for abolishing the death penalty derives from the indisputable fact that convicted persons are sometimes exonerated posthumously. Mistakes are made, and erroneous executions are irrevocable. An equally compelling argument concerns racial justice. Among all convicted murderers, a disproportionately high percentage of persons of color are sentenced to death, in all likelihood because juries and judges perceive them to be more dangerous than white murderers. But each of these lines of reasoning applies *a fortiori* to the persons eliminated by missiles launched from drones in countries where nearly everyone is a person of color, and the victims are not even charged with crimes, much less given the opportunity to defend themselves against their killers' allegation that they are evil terrorists who deserve to die. Why should a suspect have more rights within than outside the arbitrarily drawn borders of a land? If suspects have rights, then does it matter where they happen to stand? And if even convicted murderers should not be executed, as Sanders appears to believe, then how can mere suspects abroad be annihilated on the basis of purely circumstantial evidence such as SIM card data, drone video footage, and the bribed testimony of destitute, and therefore corruptible, informants on the ground?

It may be tempting to conclude from examples such as Senator Sanders that lawmakers and the citizens who elect them and pay their salaries are simple hypocrites. It is more charitable, however, and at least as plausible, that they have been trained to compartmentalize spheres of reality so effectively that what seems obviously desirable within one domain has no implications whatsoever for anywhere else. Modern people have been effectively conditioned to find nothing wrong with applying completely different standards to different spheres of reality. Their rhetoric may be absolutist, but the moral requirements upon them as individual moral persons are assumed to be a function of the context and circumstances. No less than the politicians who enthusiastically advocate for bombing abroad while decrying police brutality in the homeland, most people appear to hold a motley assortment of arguably contradictory moral beliefs, which they apply to different groups of people according to caprice and mostly determined by what they have been indoctrinated to believe, above all, by the media. In effect, modern people have developed split personalities. The innocent victims of Barack Obama's, Donald Trump's, and now Joe Biden's perpetual motion bombing campaigns do not exist in the minds of those who ordered or paid for their deaths, and are therefore excluded from all moral calculus.

The smallest sphere of morality, or moral community, comprises only oneself. At this level, morality and prudence coincide. Applying utilitarian reasoning to oneself alone yields a theory according to which one should maximize one's own happiness (or pleasure or well-being), even at the expense of others, because they lie beyond the bounds of the sphere under consideration. The next smallest sphere of morality includes one's family. After that, one's friends may be included. Then one's neighbors, one's compatriots, and, finally, humanity. No finite person can perform a full and accurate utilitarian projection of the results of his prospective action on all of humanity, and people generally consider only the short-term effects on the persons with whom they interact and of whom they are directly aware. The answer to the question "What should I do?" will vary greatly depending on whether one considers the moral community to comprise oneself (ethical egoism) or one's compatriots (nationalism) or humanity (globalism). Utilitarian-esque rhetoric pervades public discourse because it seems reasonable and sounds "moral" (rather than "selfish"), but most people either do not recognize or do not agonize over the manifest inconsistencies between what they say and what they do in the various communities in which they interact.

Avoiding altogether this morass of moral relativism, the libertarian upholds the Non-Aggression Principle (NAP), which is an easily applicable proscription: *Do not initiate — or threaten — violence against other human beings.*

Period. Do not indulge in casuistic rationalization of why it is supposedly right to bomb countries abroad when in fact there is near certainty that persons of unknown identity (and therefore not known to deserve to die) will be destroyed, no matter what the warmakers' intentions may be. Libertarians have many outspoken, virtue-signaling enemies these days, but in fact their theory is consistent, including as it does all people everywhere. If it is wrong for government agents (such as police officers) to kill suspects in the homeland, then it is equally wrong for government agents (such as drone operators) to kill suspects abroad.

Most of the federal discretionary budget goes to the military,[70] which is why utilitarian-esque defenses of federal taxation are delusive, especially in view of the twenty-year "War on Terror" fiasco. Their rhetoric notwithstanding, the policymakers who determine how much to tax citizens and where federal funds are to be allocated prioritize the interests of not humanity, nor their compatriots, but the MIC, or military-industrial-congressional-media-academic-pharmaceutical-logistics-banking complex, all tentacles of which have teams of lobbyists in Washington, D.C. In order to be completely consistent, then, it may be that libertarians should join the ranks of the war tax resisters, which is, however, easier said than done, given the harsh and coercive measures deployed by the state, again, in the name of "the greater good."

With regard to the vexing question of mandatory COVID-19 vaccination, the consistent libertarian position upholds the Nuremberg Code, according to which persons may not be experimented on without their fully informed and free consent (see Appendix B). Deceptively withholding data about the medical treatment to be imposed upon everyone everywhere (if the pro-vax camp gets their way) violates the "informed" clause of "informed consent," while coercing compliance violates the "consent" clause. In this way, the willingness of self-styled "utilitarians" to impose unwanted medical treatments upon unwilling subjects reminds us of the inherent dangers of utilitarianism in the hands of fanatics, as was clearly witnessed in Nazi Germany under the Third Reich.

10. The Con Job of the Century?

June 21, 2021
Hygiene, Colorado

Over the course of the past century, a number of truly awe-inspiring heists have been carried out by con artists, whose *modus operandi* is to exploit human frailties such as credulity, insecurity, and greed. *Con* is short for *confidence*, as the con artist must first gain the trust of his targets, after which he persuades them to hand their money over to him. A con job differs from a moral transaction between two willing, fully informed trading partners because one of the partners is deceived, and deception constitutes a form of coercion. In other words, the person being swindled is not really free. If he knew what was really going on, he would never agree to invest in the scheme.

The "Ponzi scheme"[71] was named after Charles Ponzi, who in the 1920s persuaded investors to believe that he was generating impressive profits by buying international reply coupons (IRCs) at low prices abroad and redeeming them in the United States at higher rates, the fluctuating currency market being the secret to his seemingly savvy success. In reality, Ponzi used his low-level investors' money to pay off earlier investors, to support himself, and to expand his business by luring more and more investors in. More recently, Bernie Madoff managed to abscond with billions of dollars by posing as an investment genius who could deliver sizable, indeed exceptional, returns on his clients' investments.

It is plausible that at least some of the early investors in such gambits, who are paid as promised, suppress whatever doubts may creep up in their minds as they bask in the splendor of their newfound wealth. But even those who consciously begin to grasp what is going on may turn a blind eye as the scheme grows to engulf investors who will be fleeced, having been persuaded to participate not only by the smooth-talking con artist, but also by the reported profits of previous investors. Eventually, however, the house of cards collapses, revealing the incredible but undeniable truth: there never were any investments at all. No trading ever took place, and all of the company's transactions were either deposits or withdrawals of gullible investors' cash.

Before a con artist is unmasked, nearly everyone involved plays along, either because they stand to gain, or because they truly believe. Sometimes the implications of having been wrong are simply too devastating to admit, and these same psychological dynamics operate in many other realms where most people would never suspect anything like a Ponzi scheme. It is arguable, for example, that the continuous siphoning of U.S. citizens' income to pay for misguided military interventions abroad constitutes a form of Ponzi scheme. If President George H. W. Bush had never used taxpayers' dollars to wage the First Gulf War on Iraq in 1991 and to install permanent military bases in the Middle East, then Osama bin Laden would likely never have called for jihad against the United States. If the U.S. military had not invaded Iraq in 2003, then ISIS would never have emerged and spread to Syria and beyond. Such implications are deeply unsettling, and even in the face of mounds of evidence,[72] most people prefer to cling to the official story according to which the 1991 Gulf War was necessary and just, while the terrorist attacks of September 11, 2001, were completely unprovoked, and all subsequent interventions a matter of national self-defense.

The series of bombing campaigns in the Middle East beginning in 1991 is plausibly regarded as a type of Ponzi scheme because the "investors" (taxpayers) have actually paid to make themselves worse, not better, off. Not only have the "blowback" attacks perpetrated in response to U.S. military intervention abroad killed many innocent persons, but the lives of thousands of soldiers have been, and continue to be, wrecked through dubious deployments abroad. Along with all of the blood spilled, much treasure has been lost. The more than $28 trillion national debt[73] (as of June 2021) is due in large part to the massive Pentagon budget, rubber-stamped annually by Congress, to say nothing of the many other "discretionary" initiatives claimed to be necessary in national defense. Afghanistan is a perfect example of how billions of taxpayer dollars continue to be tossed into the wind, even as the formal U.S. military presence winds down. The reason why the "War on Terror" continues on is not that it is protecting the citizens who pay for it, or helping the people of the Middle East, but because it has proved to be profitable to persons in the position to influence U.S. foreign policy.

One might reasonably assume that anyone who stands to enrich himself from government policies should be excluded from consequential deliberations over what ought to be done, and in certain realms, the quite rational concern with conflict of interest still operates to some degree. With regard to the military, however, there has been a general acquiescence by the populace to the idea that because only experts inside the system are capable of giving competent advice, they must be consulted, even when they will profit from the policies they promote, such as bombing, which invariably increases the value of stock in companies such as Raytheon. Throughout history, there has always been a push by war profiteers to promote military interventions, but Dick Cheney, who served as secretary of defense under George H. W. Bush and vice president under his son, George W. Bush, took war profiteering to an entirely new level. By privatizing many military services through the Logistics Civilian Augmentation Program (LOGCAP), Cheney effectively ushered in a period of war entrepreneurialism, beginning with Halliburton[74] (of which he was CEO from 1995 to 2000), which continues on today, making it possible for a vast nexus of subcontractors to profit from the never-ending "War on Terror," and to do so in good conscience. When more people have self-interested reasons for supporting military interventions, they become more likely to take place.

With the quelling of concerns that conflict of interest should limit the persons who advise the president on matters of foreign policy, the formal requirement that the secretary of defense be not a military officer but a civilian has been effectively dropped, with both James Mattis and Lloyd Austin easily confirmed as "exceptions" to the rule, despite the fact that, not only did both have significant financial interests in promoting war, but each also had a full career in the military before retiring and being invited to lead the Department of Defense (DOD). Military men are inclined to seek military solutions to conflict, which is undoubtedly why high-ranking officers are invited to join the boards of military companies, making Mattis and Austin textbook examples of "revolving door" appointments.

Arguably even more ruinous to the republic in the long term than the rampant conflict of interest inherent to "revolving door" appointments between the for-profit military industry and the government has been the infiltration of the military into academia, with many universities receiving large grants from the DOD for research. Academia would be a natural place for intellectual objections to the progressive militarization of society, but when scholars and scientists themselves benefit directly from Pentagon funding, they have self-interested reasons to dismiss or discredit those types of critiques — whether consciously or not — in publishing, retention, and promotion decisions. In addition to the institutional research support provided by DARPA (the Defense Advanced Research Projects Agency), successful academics may receive hefty fees as consultants for the Pentagon and its many affiliates, making them far more likely to defend the hegemon than to raise moral objections to its campaigns of mass homicide euphemistically termed "national defense."

As a result of the tentacular spread of the military, *Cui bono?* as a cautionary maxim has been replaced by *Who cares?* People seem not at all bothered by these profound conflicts of interest, and the past year has illustrated how cooption and corruption may creep easily into other realms as well. Indeed, there is a sense in which today we have two MICs: the military-industrial complex and, now, in the age of COVID-19, the medical-industrial complex. This latter development can be viewed, in part, as a consequence of the former, for in recent decades the military-industrial complex has sprouted tentacles to become the military-industrial-congressional-media-academic-pharmaceutical-logistics-banking complex. Long before COVID-19 appeared on the scene, the Veterans Administration (VA) adopted pro-Big Pharma policies, including the prescription of a vast array of psychotropic medications in lieu of "talk therapy" to treat PTSD (Post-Traumatic Stress Disorder) among veterans, and the preemptive medication of soldiers who expressed anxiety at what they were asked to do in Afghanistan and Iraq. The marked increase in the prescription of drugs to military personnel generated hefty profits for pharmaceutical firms, allowing them to expand marketing and lobbying efforts to target not only physicians but also politicians and the populace.

Since the initial marketing blitz for Prozac, beginning in 1988, the pharmaceutical industry has become an extremely powerful force in Western society, made all the more so in the United States when restrictions on direct-to-consumer advertising were lifted by the FDA (Food and Drug Administration) in 1997. Already by 2020, about 23% of Americans (nearly 77 million out of a population of 331 million) were taking psychiatric medications,[75] and those numbers appear to have increased significantly during the 2020 lockdowns,[76] which took a toll on many people's psychological well-being. As medications are prescribed more and more throughout every sector of society, drug makers exert a greater and greater influence on policy, even as the heroin/fentanyl overdose epidemic, caused directly by the aggressive marketing and rampant overprescription of narcotic painkillers, continues on.[77]

Just as the military industry is granted the benefit of the doubt on the assumption that they are helping to protect the nation, the pharmaceutical industry accrues respectability from its association with the medical profession. Who, after all, could oppose "defense" and "health"? In reality, however, for-profit weapons and drug companies are beholden not to their compatriots, nor to humanity, but to their stockholders. War and disease are profitable, while peace and health are not. The CEOs of military and pharmaceutical companies, like all businesspersons, seek to ensure that their profits increase by all means necessary, the prescription opioid epidemic being a horrific case in point.[78] Just as academics may enjoy Defense Department funding, many doctors and administrators of medical institutions today derive essential funding from drug companies and the government, whether directly or indirectly. These connections are immensely important because many politicians receive generous campaign contributions from Big Pharma, which by now has more lobbyists in Washington, D.C., than there are congresspersons, and not without reason.[79] Formulary decisions at the VA regarding the appropriateness of prescribing, for example, dangerous antipsychotic medications such as AstraZeneca's Seroquel to soldiers as sleep aids[80] are made by administrators who are political appointees, as are public health officials more generally.

With a functional Fourth Estate, it would be possible to question if not condemn the conflicts of interest operating in the for-profit military and medical realms. Unfortunately, however, we no longer have a competent press. Throughout the SARS-CoV-2 crisis, this has become abundantly clear, as alternative viewpoints on every matter of policy have been squelched, suppressed, and outright censored in the name of the truth, when there may have been ulterior motives at play. In fact, the complete quashing of any directives regarding non-vaccine therapies for mitigating the effects of COVID-19 — including Ivermectin[81] and Hydroxychloroquine[82] — may be best explained by the simple fact that FDA Emergency Use Authorization of vaccines in the United States is possible only when "there are no adequate, approved, and available alternatives," as was stated plainly on the initial specification sheets for the Pfizer[83] and Moderna[84] vaccines.

Regarding the origins of the virus, early claims by some researchers that COVID-19 may have been produced in the virology lab in Wuhan and released accidentally were swiftly dismissed as "conspiracy theories." Anyone who suggested this eminently plausible origin of the virus was immediately denounced by the media and deplatformed or censored by the Big Tech giants. "Gain-of-function" research, often funded by the military, involves making existent viruses deadlier to human beings and is said by its proponents to be necessary in order to be prepared for future natural pandemics or in the event that some enemy should use such a virus as a bioweapon. The latter is a familiar line of reasoning among military researchers, invoked also (*mutatis mutandis*) in nuclear proliferation and the military colonization of space: *We must develop the latest and greatest nuclear bombs and effect total spectrum domination of the galaxy before any other government has the chance to do so!* Many of the scientists involved in these endeavors may have the best of intentions, but that does nothing to detract from the propensity of human beings to commit errors.

In the case of COVID-19, the origin of the virus was deemed settled because Dr. Anthony Fauci, an ardent apologist for gain-of-function research and the reigning public health guru in the United States, authoritatively insisted that the transition from bats to humans came about naturally. After Fauci's pronouncement, it seemed a matter of common knowledge to "right-thinking" believers in "The Science" everywhere that the virus probably came from the wet market in Wuhan, where live animals were sold as ingredients for use in culinary delicacies such as bat soup. When the WHO looked into the matter, they appointed Peter Daszak to lead the investigation. But Daszak had in fact funded gain-of-function research by repackaging and distributing U.S. government funds through his firm EcoHealth Alliance. Needless to say, Daszak had every reason in the world to squelch any suggestion to the effect that he himself may have had something to do with the millions of deaths caused by COVID-19.

We do not yet know whether the virus had a natural or manmade origin, but if in fact U.S. taxpayer-funded research caused the pandemic and millions of deaths, then this would constitute yet another example of a government-perpetrated Ponzi scheme, rivaling and perhaps even surpassing the "War on Terror" in its negative consequences. We pay for gain-of-function research (determined by bureaucrats such as Anthony Fauci to be a good idea), and then we suffer the consequences when things go awry. Note that, just as Ponzi scheme perpetrators may begin as regular businesspersons before committing fraud, there is no need in the case of COVID-19 to invoke conspiratorial hypotheses. Many politicians who promoted and thereby helped to realize the 2003 invasion of Iraq may have been convinced that Saddam Hussein posed a grave danger to the world. Similarly, there may not have been a conscious intention on the part of anyone to let loose the

SARS-CoV-2 (COVID-19) virus on the world. After all, it's not as though incompetence among government bureaucrats is a rarity.

Whether accidentally or intentionally caused, disasters invariably pave the way for massive power grabs on the part of select persons advantageously situated. Once Iraq had been invaded, this served as the pretext for sacrificing even more blood and treasure as the quagmire intensified and spread to other countries. When the COVID-19 virus arrived on the scene, it became the pretext for a massive and abrupt transfer of wealth. Not only did much of the commerce of small businesses crushed by lockdowns migrate to companies such as Amazon and Walmart, but billions of taxpayer dollars have been poured into pharmaceutical firms.[85]

The multi-trillion dollar COVID-19 aid packages included provisions for research and development, testing, and hospitals. But the most lucrative venture in all of this frenzy has been a vaccine program with universal aspirations. The U.S. government funded the development of the COVID-19 vaccines, and now that they exist, President Biden has purchased 500 million more doses of the Pfizer product to donate to other countries.[86] The global propaganda campaign to vaccinate everyone everywhere with elixirs touted initially by their developers as having up to 95% efficacy, too, has been paid for by governments. It was unclear from the initial press releases about the spectacular new vaccines what *efficacy* actually meant, as there was a fair amount of equivocation regarding whether the treatments would confer immunity and prevent transmission of the disease, or simply lessen the severity of symptoms. After millions of persons had already been vaccinated, it emerged that the reports of 95% efficacy were at best misleading and at worst fraudulent, for the reported percentages were relative risk reduction (RRR) rates, which reflect outcomes only for the small proportion of the population vulnerable to the disease. When the rates are calculated for the general population, the vast majority of whom are not vulnerable to COVID-19, it turns out (as those who declined the vaccine had already surmised on the basis of the survival statistics) that the absolute risk reduction (ARR) rates of the Pfizer, Moderna, AstraZeneca, and Johnson & Johnson vaccines are quite low — to be precise: 0.84%, 1.2%, 1.3%, and 1.2%, respectively.[87] Nonetheless, aggressive campaigns to require vaccine passports of citizens as a condition on their resumption of normal life are everywhere on display.

A clue that the well-being of patients is not at the forefront of the minds of those running the "Vaccinate everyone!" campaign has been the encouragement of pregnant women and children to undergo vaccination, though neither group is at serious risk from the virus, and neither group was included in the trials used to secure emergency authorization. Equally surprising has been that, against all established science on immunology, the idea that persons who have already recovered from the disease must also "get the jab" has been aggressively promoted all around the globe. Judging by the media coverage, the reason for insisting that persons who were already infected with and have recovered from COVID-19 must also be vaccinated is supposed to be that people can become reinfected with the virus. That line of reasoning, however, is refuted by the statistics for reinfection. As of June 2021, out of nearly 180 million cases of COVID-19 worldwide, there were 148 confirmed cases of reinfection.[88] Studies recently published in *Nature*[89] and by the Cleveland Clinic[90] conclude that vaccination offers no benefit to previously infected persons.

In the buildup to every new war, many people who do not stand to benefit from the intervention, and may even be harmed by it, often succumb to the propaganda and enthusiastically take up the cause. In the current crisis, the false dichotomization into two exhaustive and mutually exclusive categories, the enlightened science lovers and the anti-vaxxers, is also part of a propaganda campaign. The persons who have declined vaccination, either because they already survived COVID-19 or because they prefer to wait for long-term safety data and do not believe that the possible benefits outweigh the unknown risks, are dismissed as crackpots, when in fact they are simply being prudent. Yet the media persists in propagating a misleading depiction of vaccine hesitancy in this specific case as proof of hostility toward science. This sort of polarization of the populace is, needless to say, on display during wartime as well, when anyone who dares to oppose a military intervention is depicted as a supporter of a tyrant abroad or an irrational pacifist or, when all else fails, a simple traitor.

It would be incredibly naïve to fall prey to the idea that pharmaceutical executives are somehow philanthropic, for they command enormous salaries for maximizing their stockholders' profits. In 2020, Pfizer CEO Anthony Bourla enjoyed a 17% increase in compensation, to $21 million,[91] while Moderna's CEO, Stéphane Bancel, became a billionaire.[92] The pharmaceutical industry and the military industry, despite comprising publicly traded companies, are prime examples of "crony capitalism," benefiting as they do from large infusions of cash from the government, which is allocated by bureaucrats many of whom have career and other financial interests at stake. Moreover, the funding links between the military and the public health and pharmaceutical sectors form a tangled web. Not only did the Pentagon receive a chunk of the COVID-19 rescue packages, but gain-of-function research has been paid for by military institutions. Indeed, much of the funding provided to Peter Daszak for redistribution by EcoHealth Alliance derived from the U.S. Department of Defense.[93]

Both the for-profit military and the for-profit pharmaceutical industry now use the mainstream media as a propaganda outlet to further the interests of their shareholders. Even the independent media have been infiltrated by pro-military and pro-pharma voices, which is why falsehoods such as "Saddam is in cahoots with Bin Laden and has WMD!" and "Lockdowns save lives!" are able to gain such traction among the populace. That liberty-restricting policies should be lifted only on the condition of vaccination requires people to believe that the mediation policies were both necessary and effective. But in the United States, the differences in outcomes in various states do not appear to depend on the timing or extent of lockdowns.[94] Nonetheless, just as the mass surveillance and collection of people's private data was accepted by many as a necessary part of the "War on Terror," many persons with no financial interests at stake now rally on behalf of Big Pharma for universal vaccination.

The global propaganda campaign to require people to show health papers, or a "vaccine passport," in order to participate in human society — to travel, to dine out, to shop, or to even gather together in groups — reveals that the mistakes made by a few actors are being seized upon to exert more and more control over the population. The mass surveillance of Americans was accepted by many as necessary, given the potential dangers of factional terrorism, and now, having spent more than a year whipped up by the media into a paralyzing state of fear for a virus which kills less than 1% of the persons it infects, many citizens appear willing to accept what influential globalists have been insisting must be "the new normal." This is a grave mistake.

It is too early to know how this unprecedented chapter in human history will end, but the trends are not encouraging. With countries continuing their serial lockdowns and travel restrictions, along with masking, testing, and quarantine requirements, they deepen the divisions already on display, making it seem more likely that some form of apartheid state with totalitarian qualities will emerge. Does any government have the right to force its citizens to undergo a medical treatment of which, according to all available statistical data, they have no need? Why are universities requiring vaccination as a condition of enrollment and employment? Why are more doctors not rising up to challenge the aggressive push to vaccinate everyone everywhere with an experimental treatment? There is no medical basis whatsoever for requiring previously infected persons to undergo vaccination, which has never been demanded in the case of any other disease.

What is at stake is not merely inconvenience, and the solution is not, as some liberty lovers have suggested (if only facetiously), to acquire a forged vaccine passport. We should reject in the most categorical of terms the very idea that anyone anywhere should be required to prove his health status to anyone else, and that anyone anywhere should be compelled to undergo a medical treatment against his own will — whatever his reasons may be. One's medical choices affect one's health, well-being, and body, which no government can be said to own. To relinquish one's right to one's own body is to render oneself the property of a tyrannical state. If citizens permit the government to strip them of their right to make decisions about how to lead their very own lives, then they will have been fleeced far worse than the victims of the most mercenary Ponzi scheme, having paid with their freedom for their future enslavement.

11. How Not to Treat Human Beings as Moral Persons

July 16, 2021
Ogden, Utah

Immanuel Kant, an eighteenth-century German philosopher, famously espoused the following maxim of morality:

> Act in such a way that you treat humanity… never merely as a means to an end, but always at the same time as an end.

The terms of this principle, a formulation of what Kant calls the "Categorical Imperative," are rather abstract, but he also provided a more practical test for determining whether a prospective action is morally permissible or not:

> Act only according to that maxim whereby you can at the same time will that it should become a universal law.

According to Kant, violations of this formulation of the Categorical Imperative embroil one in a "practical contradiction." It is not immediately obvious what he means by this, which is why his œuvre continues to be a lively subject of debate among professional philosophers. Those sympathetic with Kant's general outlook have sometimes drawn parallels to more familiar principles of the major religions, including the Golden Rule:

> Do unto others as you would have them do unto you.

Even without having studied philosophical ethics, many people will nonetheless aver that when we talk colloquially about someone *using* another person, the implication is that it is immoral. Excellent examples include notorious "black widows" (and widowers), who murder their spouses in order to gain possession of their wealth. In fact, every case of mercenarily motivated murder would seem likewise to violate Kant's Categorical Imperative — and the Golden Rule. The idea of not using people solely as the means to our selfish ends coheres rather well with commonsense morality and is embedded in the legal systems of modern Western democracies.

Much ink has been spilled over the past few centuries by scholars in rejecting Kant's deontological theory in favor of more practical — teleological or consequentialist — approaches such as utilitarianism, according to which one should always act so as to maximize the happiness or pleasure (or *utility*, as John Stuart Mill and Jeremy Bentham termed it) of the greatest number of people. According to utilitarianism, no action is excluded from the outset, because one must determine what its consequences will be in order to know whether it is right or wrong. If a black widower donates his miserly wife's estate to help people in dire need, then a strict utilitarian might in fact deem the murder (intentional, premeditated act of homicide) to be the right course of action. More generally, if by sacrificing one person or a small number of persons one will thereby save millions of morally equivalent others, staunch utilitarians will insist that the sacrifice not only can but *should* be made.

Quasi-utilitarian reasoning is found frequently among calls for wars of so-called humanitarian intervention, which promoters claim will save many more people than doing nothing, even though there will invariably be some "collateral damage" victims who die as a direct result of the bombing itself. The outcomes of modern bombing campaigns never reflect the sunny forecasts of those who set the intervention machine in motion, but even if they did, this rationalization for "humanitarian intervention" assumes that killing and letting die are morally equivalent, a position which is rejected within the bounds of civil society.[95] Except in rare cases, involving persons with special obligations of care, such as physicians and parents, we do not regard permitting people to die as the moral equivalent of killing them.

The ongoing mess in the Middle East[96] shows how wrong the prognosticators were when they claimed that the invasion of Iraq in 2003 would be swift and simple, ushering in an era of peace and democracy for Iraqis, who instead went from suffering under the rule of a despot to living in a chaotic and deadly environment in which their security and quality of life were severely degraded. The state of Libya a decade after the 2011 bombing campaign and the ouster of Muammar Gaddafi is another striking example of how wrong self-styled "humanitarian interventionists" can be about the consequences of their "well-intended" programs of homicide.

One reason why hawks reach so facilely for utilitarian rationalizations for their wars may be that in this approach to normative morality there is no need to reflect seriously upon the plight of individual soldiers. The end justifies the means, and, yes, that will include the sacrifice of some young persons in the prime of their lives. In galvanizing support for invading and bombing other countries, the effects on soldiers — the thousands who may be physically maimed or killed, and the many thousands more who may be psychologically wrecked by the experience — are not mentioned at all because they are not recognized as real until after the fact, and then only by some. Indeed, the U.S. military itself has repeatedly and systematically denied responsibility for injuries to soldiers — caused by the spraying of Agent Orange in Vietnam, the bombing of chemical facilities in the First Gulf War, the use of burn pits during the occupations, etc. — even in the face of overwhelming evidence that the soldiers were harmed not by the enemy but as a direct result of their own military leadership's callous disregard for the well-being of troops. In those cases where culpability was finally acknowledged, it took years of activism in order for this to happen.

Utilitarian-esque reasoning is quite versatile and is readily invoked in debates on a variety of other military matters as well. Opposition to military conscription, for example, can be made on the purely utilitarian grounds that coerced soldiers are unlikely to fight as effectively as volunteers. Accordingly, whenever soldiers are forced to fight, rather than invited to do so, the outcomes will likely be worse than they would otherwise have been. In World War I, this problem was "solved" by sending wave after wave of young men to their deaths, effectively expending them as cannon fodder.

The Kantian reason for opposing military conscription, whereby unwilling persons are coerced to fight, to kill, and possibly to die in wars over which they have no say, differs markedly from the utilitarian perspective. Efficacy, far from being morally decisive, is in fact irrelevant in the Kantian moral framework. What is wrong with conscription is not that it will have negative consequences, but that such soldiers are treated merely as the means to the ends of political elites. Alongside draftees, many a volunteer soldier has been squandered as cannon fodder, but so long as he freely entered into the Faustian bargain of agreeing to kill and risking his own life in exchange for employment, benefits, etc., then he is not being *used* in the same sense in which every drafted soldier is.

Now, there are good reasons for thinking that war as a means to conflict resolution is at least irrational, if not intrinsically immoral, because no one should ever agree to kill complete strangers at the behest of war promoters, many of whom stand to profit from their programs — whether financially or politically, and often both. But as a result in part of the long-entrenched myth of heroic warriors who take up arms everywhere and only in the name of "justice" — *so long as they are on our side!* — wars do continue to be waged and fought, victims slain, and soldiers sacrificed. Relative to *that* world, delusional though it may be, forcing persons to take up arms is still worse than allowing them to do so.[97]

As shocking as it may seem, twentieth-century soldiers were experimented on in a variety of contexts, under what appears to have been the assumption that they had already signed their lives over to the military, *so why not?* During the 1991 Gulf War and in the following years, U.S. soldiers were required to be vaccinated against Anthrax using a yet-to-be-approved (by the FDA) pharmaceutical product which caused significant bodily harm to some of the troops.[98] As a result of the Anthrax vaccine fiasco, soldiers are no longer required to undergo experimental treatments, including the emergency authorized COVID-19 vaccines, which have yet to receive full FDA approval. Needless to say, the pharmaceutical and biotech companies involved are doing everything within their means to obtain an early approval so that the vaccines can be mandated by law in a variety of contexts, including the military.

More generally, the current COVID-19 crisis provides a refractive lens through which to distinguish the two very different ways of conceiving of morality, the deontological (as exemplified by Kantianism) and the teleological (as exemplified by utilitarianism). Human experimentation, such as the mass vaccination programs currently underway, is carried out under the utilitarian assumption that the sacrifice of a few will ultimately save millions of lives. Every medical treatment, even those which have received years of testing and full FDA approval, has negative outlier effects on a small portion of the population, and it is purely a matter of misfortune to be one of the persons who ends up being harmed rather than helped. No one has been singled out for harm, so the situation is similar to a lottery where most people win the prize — in this case immunity or, at the very least, better prospects for survival in the case of infection — but a small percentage do not.

The Vaccine Adverse Effect Reporting System (VAERS) database[99] catalogues the reported harms caused by vaccines, and in the case of COVID-19, these have included myocarditis, severe allergic or immune reactions, and Bell's Palsy, among other possible effects, up to and including death. That these vaccines are being distributed in an ongoing experimental trial is underscored by the fact that the specification sheets for recipients and caregivers were recently updated to reflect the incidence of heart disease as a rare but possible side effect. That risk was not recognized in the early, much smaller, trials, nor in the initial roll-out to elderly persons, but became clear only upon the vaccination of younger persons, who would ordinarily not have heart troubles, as older persons sometimes do.

So long as patients are properly informed of the potential dangers, if ever so slim, to their health and well-being, then it is their prerogative to incur risks in exchange for the prospective benefits of vaccination, should they deem this to be the proper course of action for themselves. In other words, the case may be viewed as similar to a fully informed person who agrees to enlist in the military, even while knowing the risks involved. There are, however, some curious factors in the present case which together suggest that nothing like morality is driving the quest for universal vaccination. Most obviously, a heavy-handed and ubiquitous propaganda campaign is being used to persuade persons to believe that it is somehow wrongheaded, ignorant, and/or selfish not to agree to serve as a subject in an experimental trial for a treatment of which many of them have no need, given their prospects for survival even without the vaccine.

Under normal circumstances, individual persons, so long as they are mentally competent, are deemed the appropriate authorities about which treatments to undertake in efforts to protect themselves and enjoy good health — or not. Free people are also permitted to smoke, eat junk food, avoid exercise, consume alcohol as they please, and engage in risk-taking activities such as rock-climbing or surfing in dangerous waters at their caprice, even though any of these behaviors may result in premature death. In the current crisis, we have seen endless exhortations to universal vaccination from figureheads such as President Biden and Vice President Harris, both of whom recently emoted on Twitter: "Get vaccinated, or wear a mask until you do!" Such sweeping prescriptions on the part of persons with no information about the individual patients whom they are sternly enjoining to undergo treatment would be a clear violation of medical ethics, if in fact Biden and Harris were physicians, which of course they are not.

Competent medical professionals do not issue blanket prescriptions to be followed uniformly and mindlessly by all possible patients. The particular circumstances of particular patients call for particular treatments to be undertaken — or not. Sound medical advice derives from a licensed professional who is familiar with the condition and circumstances of the patient in question. There is no prescription applicable simultaneously to infants, toddlers, adolescents, young adults, pregnant women, middle-aged persons, and nonagenarians, because their bodily conditions are completely different. Moreover, even within each partitioned category, a wide range of variation exists. Some people (whatever their age) are obese, while others are not. Some people have smoked or continue to smoke, while others do not. Some suffer allergies, while others do not. It is nothing short of incompetent to suggest that any treatment should be applied in a one-size-fits-all fashion, as is being done in the propaganda campaigns for the COVID-19 vaccines. Far worse than offering people incompetent (because ill-informed) medical advice, however, would be to force them to comply with mandatory edicts derived from incompetent medical advice.

An overzealous judge (Richard Frye) in Ohio recently sentenced three persons convicted in his court of law to COVID-19 vaccination,[100] which would seem to be a flagrant violation of civil rights. Certainly, the punishment cannot possibly be said to fit the crime, because it is completely irrelevant to it — to any crime, as a matter of fact. The judge explained his decision in the following terms, "It occurred to me that some of these folks needed to be encouraged not to procrastinate," demonstrating only that he has no business residing over any court of law, for he has decided to use the courtroom as his personal pulpit, legislating from the bench in the most obnoxious of ways. One of the criminals, Sylvaun Latham, was offered the choice of COVID-19 vaccination plus a one-year term of probation or else a five-year term of probation. In other words, his liberty to conduct himself as he pleases was tethered by the judge to his willingness to serve now as a subject in an ongoing experimental trial of the COVID-19 vaccine, which is not scheduled to end until 2023.

To require convicts to serve as subjects in experimental trials for drug treatments for which they may or may not have any need is tantamount to making them the property of the state and their lives the prerogative of the state to risk and even to sacrifice. (See *The Imitation Game* [2014], a film directed by Morten Tyldum, for the tragic story of Alan Turing in Britain.) This is a very different scenario from voluntary conscription, whereby fully informed persons agree in exchange for remuneration to risk their own lives and well-being. But soldiers who volunteer to fight for their country do not simultaneously agree to serve as pharmaceutical company guinea pigs, which is why forced experimentation on soldiers, too, is wrong. As difficult as it may be to believe, we have now entered an era in which so-called public health experts who support mandatory vaccination are galvanizing judges to conduct themselves in the manner of the officials of the Third Reich. During that deplorable episode of history, judges regularly sentenced persons to sterilization, and many persons were used in human experimentation against their own will.

The most important conclusion of the Nuremberg court regarding human experimentation was this:

> The voluntary consent of the human subject is absolutely essential. This means that the person involved should have legal capacity to give consent; should be so situated as to be able to exercise free power of choice, without the intervention of any element of force, fraud, deceit, duress, overreaching, or other ulterior form of constraint or coercion; and should have sufficient knowledge and comprehension of the elements of the subject matter involved as to enable him to make an understanding and enlightened decision.

Extorting convicts to undergo experimental vaccination in exchange for shorter prison or probation sentences clearly violates this Nuremberg court finding (see Appendix B). Indeed, every case of "force, fraud, deceit, duress, overreaching, or other ulterior form of constraint or coercion" to undergo medical treatment is also a violation.

Going even farther than the Ohio judge who imposed vaccine sentences upon convicted criminals, the government of France is effectively criminalizing those who refuse to participate in the vaccine trials. On July 12, 2021 (ironically two days before Bastille Day), President Emmanuel Macron announced that proof of vaccination will be required in social venues, on public transport, and, in some cases, to remain gainfully employed.[101] By denying persons the right to use public transportation, or even to work, the French government is especially targeting poor people, for wealthy people have private cars and do not need to work. But all "non-compliant" French citizens are being punished as though they committed crimes, when in fact they have every right in the world to decide which medical treatments to undergo and which to decline. These measures effectively transform French society into an everted prison in which everyone who refuses to offer his body for use in an experimental trial has his liberties curtailed as though he were an incarcerated criminal who was convicted of a crime. In effect, everyone who declines the experimental vaccine is being put under house arrest.

In the United States, some businesses are requiring vaccination of their employees, and quite a few universities are requiring vaccination of both employees and students, even though the chance of deleterious, life-changing, or even deadly vaccine side effects may for some cohorts (such as young males) be greater than the chance of death should they become infected with COVID-19. It is nothing short of extortion to threaten people with extremely negative consequences should they not volunteer to serve in an experimental trial for a drug/device of which they have no need. *You want to finish your college degree? You want to remain gainfully employed? Then roll up your sleeve!* And yet a disturbing number of otherwise apparently rational people support these initiatives, at least judging by their comportment on social media. (Note that there are many bot farms operating on this front as well, and whether they are being paid for by governments or the companies who stand to profit is unclear.)

On July 6, 2021, President Biden announced his administration's intention to send vaccine promoters door-to-door to persuade those who have not already complied to change their mind.[102] The assumption behind this "folksy" approach of "community outreach" is that people who decline vaccination are ill-informed, but with the appropriate amount of friendly banter, they will recognize the error of their ways. The problem, however, is that, *pace* Anthony Fauci, "The Science" has not spoken yet. The information censored and dismissed as disinformation by the media and those who parrot its every proclamation includes hypotheses, theories, and bald facts which do not support the reigning narrative and suggest that it may well be false. While appealing to a "community outreach" spirit, Biden also likened this initiative to a "war-time" effort and called willingness to be vaccinated "patriotic," the insinuation being that declining vaccination is unpatriotic.

Preposterously, given the thousands of breakthrough cases of persons fully vaccinated but who have contracted COVID-19 anyway, the so-called vaccines may not effectively prevent transmission but only mitigate symptoms — which is what they were designed to do. The shots offer a very slim risk reduction (ARR, or absolute risk reduction, of ~1%) to most people, because most people are not vulnerable to COVID-19, making it far from obvious that there is any reason for them to undergo an experimental treatment.[103] Yet facts appear incapable of slowing the propaganda machine set in motion more than a year ago, and vaccine proselytizers persist in haranguing even the millions of already recovered persons to roll up their sleeves.

The global propaganda campaign has been so relentless and vast that those who decline vaccination, as in France, stand to have their liberties severely curtailed by government bureaucrats the world over who cling tenaciously to disinformation about the supposed superiority of vaccine immunity over natural immunity, despite numerous studies demonstrating the robustness of the latter and mountains of evidence that social mitigation measures have no effect on outcomes from place to place. Strikingly, if the vaccines do not prevent infection, but only diminish symptoms, then millions of vaccinated persons should be expected to fall into the supposed class of "asymptomatic carriers" and be more likely to transmit the virus to other people once they stop wearing masks and practicing social distancing — at least according to the religious tenets of the Branch Covidians.

As in every other case when quasi-utilitarian rationalizations have been trotted out in support of policies which will destroy some persons' lives, no one has any idea what the long-term effects of the vaccination programs will be. To pretend otherwise is to lie and, in Kant's view, to deceive and thereby to treat the persons in question merely as means, not as ends in themselves. To treat people as moral persons is to grant them the dignity of being able to inform themselves, assess the facts, and come to their own conclusions about how best to conduct their own lives, up to and including which medical procedures to undertake.

Anyone who agrees that it is wrong to use people solely as a means should be wary of pseudo-utilitarian propaganda, above all when the self-styled utilitarians have nothing to lose and something to gain. That there exist today people who are rallying for forced vaccination by the government of the very people whom the government supposedly serves reveals, once again, as many historical episodes attest, how frightened people can be persuaded to support objectively abhorrent policies, sacrifice their fellow human beings, and renounce their very own rights.

When Biden's Pfizer minions show up at your doorstep, let us hope that they do not in their missionary fervor undertake to vaccinate you without your consent. Just as the cases of President Macron and Judge Frye illustrate, for fanatics convinced of their intellectual superiority and moral righteousness, the end always justifies the means. The danger of this political climate for free people cannot be overestimated. Given the length and range of the COVID-19 vaccine propaganda campaigns, which have completely saturated the mainstream media, there is some reason for suspecting that readily available forms of forced vaccination may be nearer than we think, given the willingness of state authorities such as judges and presidents to criminalize the refusal to serve as a subject in a pharmaceutical product trial.

That Biden has claimed to be on a "wartime" footing *vis-à-vis* COVID-19, and the Pentagon itself recently held a "war game" specifically addressing the COVID-19 crisis, certainly does not bode well for the future of free people. The technology already exists to be able to vaccinate the unwilling using aerosol sprays which could be delivered by automated drone swarms. As horrifyingly dystopic as that possibility may sound, we already know from their many military misadventures abroad that government officials are ready and willing to use any and all of the implements in their arsenal in achieving their aims, and they have no problem ignoring altogether the moral personhood of their victims.

12. Throttling the Truth: Why the Case of Julian Assange Is More Important Than Ever

August 24, 2021
Austin, Texas

In a world with a functional Fourth Estate, the case of Julian Assange would be on the front page of major newspapers every day. Instead, it has been all but blacked out. Perhaps this makes sense, given that the *raison d'être* of WikiLeaks, according to its founder, was to provide the public with important news which is omitted by the mainstream media outlets. To defend WikiLeaks in a sustained way would be for network news channels and syndicated newspapers to acknowledge, at least tacitly, that they have been coopted by the government, as critics have long maintained. Nonetheless, the unwillingness of truth-driven journalists to say more about what is going on is puzzling and suggests that the situation is far worse than we may imagine. The future of press freedom is at stake and with it the very possibility of dissent.

In some ways, the U.S. government's quest to silence Assange has already succeeded, for the founder of WikiLeaks is no longer having any effect on the world, and he has had very little effect since 2018, when his Internet access was cut off. From 2012 to 2019, Assange lived in the Ecuadorian Embassy in London, having sought asylum there in order to avoid persecution by the U.S. government. He was wrenched from his safe haven in 2019, when the government of Ecuador stopped protecting him and permitted the British government forcibly to remove him from the premises. This appears to have been a case of bribery or threat, and most likely both, given the well-established modes of "persuasion" used by the U.S. superpower to bend lesser powers to its will. Whatever ultimately precipitated his ejection from the embassy, Assange was taken away by agents of the United Kingdom and placed in Belmarsh prison, where he remains today, awaiting the court's decision on whether to extradite him so that he can be made to stand trial in the United States on charges of espionage.

Assange, an Australian citizen, published troves of secret documents stolen by whistleblowers who wished to illuminate what they took to be malfeasance, both in the Global War on Terror and in the DNC's

(Democratic National Committee's) efforts to determine the outcome of the Democratic presidential primary election in 2016. I suspect that, if the extradition quest succeeds, the death knell for Julian Assange will have been not the dissemination of war-related materials, such as the shocking "Collateral Murder" video[104] showing Reuters journalists "neutralized" in Iraq by soldiers hovering above in an Apache helicopter, but the revelation that the progressive candidate Bernie Sanders never stood a chance against the pre-selected nominee of Democratic Party elites, Hillary Clinton.

I say this because despite the fact that Assange's asylum at the Ecuadorian Embassy was abruptly ended under President Trump, and may well have been a cynical and primarily political ploy to discredit further the already discredited Russian collusion narrative, the Biden administration continues to pursue Assange just as ruthlessly. According to the Russian collusion hoax, which dominated U.S. political discourse for more than three entire years and continues to be discussed by some pundits still today, Trump was elected the President of the United States in 2016 *only* because of the Russians. Trump's election had nothing whatsoever to do with the fact that Hillary Clinton was an abysmal candidate who haughtily called half the nation "deplorable," nor because she was a hawk who rallied for the disastrous 2003 invasion of Iraq, nor because she was instrumental in persuading President Obama to bomb Libya, among other foreign policy disasters to her credit. Just as I doubt that President Biden will pardon whistleblower Daniel Hale,[105] because doing so would tarnish the image of Barack Obama by acknowledging that he lied about the drone program, I doubt that Biden/Harris will drop the charges against Assange, who is blamed by all self-styled right-minded Democrats for the election of Donald Trump.

Whoever shared the DNC email trove with WikiLeaks (whether Russian trolls or Seth Rich, the DNC staffer murdered in Washington, D.C., on July 10, 2016 — or perhaps someone else altogether), the missives clearly revealed to Bernie Sanders voters that they had been played. All of their hours of volunteer work, all of their hard-earned cash donated in small sums to a campaign doomed to fail from the start, were obviously for naught. There can be little doubt that some Sanders supporters declined to vote at all in 2016 after discovering in Clinton campaign chairman John Podesta's emails what had been going on behind the scenes at the DNC. Thousands of registered Democrats left the party in what they hashtagged as a #DEMEXIT protest, and some among them went even so far as to vote for

Donald Trump. For this, Assange will never be forgiven by millions of people, some of whom continue to suffer from Trump Derangement Syndrome (TDS) and persist in blaming the Russians for every catastrophe under the sun. Rational people recognize, of course, that if the DNC had not rigged the election, then there would be no reason for their voters to be angered by the primary result. Resolute "I'm With Her" Hillary Clinton supporters are not bothered in the least by the behind-closed-doors shenanigans of the DNC, but only by the fact that they were made public by WikiLeaks.

Assange also shared with the public evidence of U.S. war crimes, so one reason his case is rarely mentioned by anyone in the mainstream media is simply that war coverage is slanted to support the U.S. military. Viewed as a simple market-driven problem, the major news channels today are primarily in the business of infotainment rather than journalism, and it seems unlikely that pointing out that taxpayers fund the murder of innocent people abroad could do anything but lower ratings. The networks are obviously more interested in audience satisfaction than truth, as the case of Rachel Maddow illustrates. A judge recently ruled that Maddow is not a journalist but a liberal activist,[106] who offers hyperbole in place of facts and "distorts reality." This, however, is supposedly fine because her viewers are expected to know that she is not reporting the news but sharing her own often emotional views. During the Trump years, the author of *Drift: The Unmooring of American Military Power* (2012)[107] somehow lost the journalistic plot to become Hillary Clinton's arch apologist, ironically comporting herself in a manner not unlike Alex Jones and abandoning altogether her former role as an antiwar critic. Needless to say, Maddow, in contrast to Jones, has not been deplatformed across the Big Tech outlets and denounced as a lunatic, for she, unlike Jones, is a *useful* sensationalist, who has come dutifully to serve the establishment.

There was a time, years ago, when Julian Assange was still being discussed quite a bit in the mainstream media, and that initial, propaganda-riddled coverage seems to have got lodged in people's minds. In my travels around the world, I have been surprised by the responses of people in completely different places to my questions about the founder of WikiLeaks. Anecdotally, I can report that there are apparently intelligent, reasonably well-informed people, not only in the United States but also in the United Kingdom, New Zealand, and even Assange's country of citizenship, Australia, who believe that he is an underhanded, morally despicable criminal. This they take to have been demonstrated by the fact that Assange was summoned back to Sweden to answer allegations of rape some years ago but "bolted," as his critics characterize it, rather than confront his accusers back in 2012.

Nearly a decade after Assange took refuge in the Ecuadorian embassy, it no longer seems to matter to many of those same people that Swedish authorities abandoned the Assange case for lack of evidence to sustain an indictment. The initial portrait painted of Assange, in a very effective discreditation effort, as someone who cowardly evaded justice by hiding out in the embassy, looms larger in many people's minds than the crimes which he exposed. Needless to say, this morally unsavory portrait was made even uglier to Hillary Clinton Democrats after the leak of DNC emails which most likely did contribute to Donald Trump's election in 2016, regarded by so many as "unthinkable."

The Assange haters, in clinging to the image created for them by the media, are either unwilling or unable to consider rational explanations, such as simple prudence, for Assange's decision to protect himself through seeking political asylum. To offer only one of many possible examples, consider the plight of Michael Hastings, one of the most effective antiwar journalists to have emerged on the scene in the twenty-first century and whose work actually ended the career of General Stanley McChrystal.[108] Hastings died under strange circumstances in a single-car automobile accident on June 18, 2013, shortly after having told friends that he was being pursued somehow by the FBI, and also that someone had been tinkering with his car. Suggestions to the effect that there may have been foul play involved were swiftly dismissed, and Hastings has by now been forgotten by all but a few "conspiracy theorists." But it is a fact (disclosed by none other than WikiLeaks) that single-car accidents are a specialty of the CIA, and Hastings had picked fights with people in very high places. Indeed, at the time of his death, Hastings was working on an exposé of Obama's lethal drone czar, John Brennan, who had been confirmed as CIA director on March 8, 2013. The Los Angeles Police Department (LAPD) declined to investigate the case, and Hastings's wife, Elise Jordan (a former speechwriter for Condoleezza Rice, improbably enough), went out on the media circuit to insist that the death was an accident.

Whatever may or may not have been done to Hastings, the point is that Julian Assange, being acutely aware of what the CIA and its affiliates were capable of doing, acted altogether prudently in protecting himself by seeking refuge in the Ecuadorian embassy, and remaining there up until he was forcibly removed. The "Collateral Murder" video footage, after all, depicted the execution of journalists. Even more ominously, Obama's expansion of the drone program effectively normalized extrajudicial killing, formerly known as "assassination," of non-citizens and citizens alike. From the cases of Anwar al-Awlaki; his son, Abdulrahman al-Awlaki; and Samir Khan (editor and publisher of *Inspire* magazine), all killed in 2011, there can no longer be any doubt that the U.S. government is willing to kill even its own citizens with no due process whatsoever.[109]

Before being muted and sequestered, Julian Assange, like both Michael Hastings and Anwar al-Awlaki, was a very public and vocal opponent of U.S. military interventions in the Middle East. Once in the Ecuadorian embassy, Assange and his lawyers were spied upon,[110] which surely counts as evidence that his concern for his own safety was sound. Added to that, according to his defense team, there were discussions among paid Spanish operatives about ending Assange's life while he was under asylum.[111] Nonetheless, Assange, who has been kept in Belmarsh prison with very little interaction with anyone for more than two years, is being treated as though *he* were a convicted criminal.

On July 7, 2021, the U.K. High Court ruled that the U.S. government could continue its quest for extradition, and on August 11, 2021, a judge ruled that Assange will remain in prison while the U.S. government is permitted to expand the grounds for its appeal, having raised doubts about the mental health pretext used in the January 4, 2021, court judgment according to which extradition to a supermax prison in the United States might lead to Assange's suicide. What is undeniably a concerted effort to muffle the founder of WikiLeaks is succeeding, for he continues to be wholly consumed with the matter of his own survival. This despite the obvious violation of procedure through spying on him and his lawyers, and despite the fact that Sigurdur Ingi Thordarson, a key witness in the U.S. case against Assange, revealed in an Icelandic newspaper that he had fabricated his story in exchange for immunity offered to him by U.S. authorities.[112]

The U.S. government wishes to try Assange, under their expansive interpretation of the 1917 Espionage Act, for having illegally obtained and disseminated top secret U.S. government documents. But surely Assange has neither a legal nor a moral duty to support the government of the United

States, least of all when he believes that it regularly commits war crimes, evidence of which he has made public and for which he is now being persecuted. As many critics have insisted, to claim that Assange violated U.S. law through publishing documents obtained and shared by whistleblowers sets a very dangerous precedent, expanding the power of the state to the point of being able to stifle dissent and prevent journalists from reporting on war crimes committed by governments anywhere. This is a step onto a totalitarian slope, allowing only the state propaganda department to determine what constitute the facts and allowing the government both to deny and to hide all evidence of the government's own crimes, such as those detailed in the Afghanistan War Diary[113] and the Iraq War Diary[114] published by WikiLeaks.

After twenty years of squandered blood and treasure, the U.S. war in Afghanistan ended unceremoniously with the Taliban taking over the country, demonstrating once again, as the saying goes, that Afghanistan is "the place where empires go to die." Predictably, the major networks have continued to tap the usual suspects, the incompetent war architects themselves, to criticize not the war itself but the manner in which it was ended. While foreign policy experts seem at the moment to be consumed with an ugly blame game, I suspect that the timing of the U.S. withdrawal had more to do with other, more ambitious projects in the works, and in no way reflects an abandonment by political elites of their imperial aims. For it is becoming increasingly clear that there is a vigorous and well-orchestrated effort, in countries all around the globe, to create a different sort of world altogether, one where places such as Afghanistan no longer matter much at all.

Placing the case of Assange into the broader context of ongoing efforts to squelch dissent, it is noteworthy that the Biden administration press secretary, Jen Psaki, recently revealed, in a display of open scorn for the First Amendment to the U.S. Constitution, that the government is "working closely with Facebook" to stop the dissemination of what they regard as misinformation.[115] But Psaki herself is open to charges of disinformation, not only about the COVID-19 vaccines, about which she parrots Fauci, claiming a mythical "The Science" as her source of knowledge, but also whenever she speaks about Biden's predecessor. In an exchange with a reporter over negative vaccine messaging by Biden before becoming president, Psaki quipped, "I would note that at the time, just for context, the former president was also suggesting people inject versions of poison into their veins to cure COVID. So I think that's a relevant point." There is no film or document in which Trump tells people to inject themselves with poison or to drink bleach, because he never did.[116]

The Biden Ministry of Propaganda continues nonetheless to keep these tropes alive just as surely as the Bush team continued to pretend that Saddam Hussein really did have WMD and was somehow in cahoots with Al Qaeda, even as it became increasingly obvious that neither was true. The situation has become far more perilous now, however, for the very future of the republic. The government has long worked closely with the mass media news outlets, especially to promote war, but the very possibility of whistleblowing is in danger of being altogether eliminated as the government works with the Big Tech companies to censor so-called disinformation on the only available alternative news source, the Internet. Already in 2021, the U.S. government seized entire websites in Iran, and there is little reason to think that they will stop there. After all, one country's cyberattack is another country's act of national defense.[117]

In her press conference, Psaki was referring to "misinformation" about COVID-19, meaning reports in conflict with the administration's own narrative, but by the same logic, there could no longer be any dissent from the misadventures of the U.S. military, no matter what they did. Convicting Assange as a spy would likely put an end to what small amount of true journalism continues on today, cementing the current substitution of propaganda for news, with the government granting the government itself the right to black out sites such as WikiLeaks altogether. Before sermons by Anwar al-Awlaki were removed from the Internet,[118] he was "convicted" of terrorism in the public eye by extrajudicial state execution. If Assange were convicted in a court of law of espionage, then some in the government could be expected to feel justified in erasing every trace of his work from the world.

If the Internet, along with the mainstream media, comes to be completely controlled by the government, then dissent will be impossible, and a formerly democratic society will have been transformed into a totalitarian system, where oligarchs determine what may and may not be said, and those who demur are criminalized, not for violent or fraudulent acts, but for disagreeing with "the official story" and standing up for the truth. We have seen how redefining "offense" as "defense" and "bombing" as "humanitarian intervention" were cynical but highly successful ploys to promote the war machine. Those who dare to dissent, like Assange, and manage to do it effectively, are discredited and deplatformed, by hook or by crook.

In the current COVIDystopic climate, even credentialed scientists and doctors are permitted only to parrot the decrees of the government's small committee of policymakers with clear financial ties to the pharmaceutical industry. When they dare to demur, backing up their dissent with data-based research, they are deplatformed. Astonishingly, it has become official government policy in many places around the world that healthy people can be criminalized as public menaces and citizens required, on pain of loss of civil liberties, to serve as subjects in experimental trials for medical treatments of which they have no need.

Under Obama, the presumption of suspect innocence was perversely inverted to become a presumption of guilt and used as the pretext for executing thousands of persons located outside areas of active hostility.[119] Now we are witnessing an inversion of presumed health to sickness, with citizens being required to demonstrate their vaccination status in order to go about their daily lives. We have seen over a matter of mere months political leaders go from attempting to bribe citizens to undergo experimental vaccination in exchange for lottery tickets, cash payments, and free food, to criminalizing their very attempt to conduct their lives peaceably in civil society by attending public events, dining out, using public transport, visiting museums, or going shopping.

The Department of Homeland Security recently listed "Opposition to COVID Measures" as one of its "Potential Terror Threats." What happens next? We know from history that once groups of people are convincingly portrayed by the government as despicable criminals and pariahs, then there is no limit to what "good people" will do to see that they be eliminated, and those who have freely declined the COVID-19 vaccines are now being punished in the cities of Paris, New York, Los Angeles, and New Orleans, where they are no longer permitted to participate in society. The most frightening aspect of the propaganda campaign currently underway is that it has been propagated through easy-to-parrot soundbites (such as "Listen to The Science!") which many people, in states of total self-deception, proclaim from the hilltops against what they take to be the unwashed, unvaxxed, unmasked, and ignorant enemy. So convinced are compliant citizens by now of their moral righteousness that many of them will not even engage in discussions with those who disagree.

The revelations of Julian Assange, Chelsea (then Bradley) Manning, and Daniel Hale demonstrated for all to see the government's assertion of the right to kill anyone anywhere, without indictment or trial, on whatever grounds it deems sufficient. Assassination is certainly the most direct and facile way of dealing with dissidents who are articulate enough to defend themselves in a court of law. Anwar al-Awlaki, for example, was able to convey clear, antiwar, anti-imperialist objections to the U.S. government's fiascos in the Middle East. Rather than allow him to pose an intellectual threat to the official story, by having him stand trial in a court of law, al-Awlaki was summarily silenced for all time through incineration by lethal drone.

Perhaps, then, no one should be surprised by the increasingly aggressive attempts by Western governments to coerce citizens to submit to experimental medical treatments, even while death has been acknowledged to be one of a number of documented side effects. The latest spec sheets for the Pfizer[120] and Moderna[121] vaccines now include a full paragraph warning about the danger of myocarditis, but the propaganda campaign to vaccinate young persons at nearly no risk from COVID-19 plows ahead with the CDC now recommending a third "booster" shot for everyone who has already received two shots, regardless of age or health condition.

As data continues to be amassed, more and more research studies are appearing to vindicate the "quacks" who disagreed early on with the reigning global public health narrative. These studies may be ignored by the Biden administration's Ministry of Propaganda, but we must patiently await the day when the fear of the virus no longer propels people to follow the government's arbitrary *diktats* blindly, nor to pressure their neighbors into doing the same. Public health officials, being political appointees, will not save the world from what looks at this point to be an inexorable march toward totalitarianism.

Our last, best hope lies in the courts. We must mount lawsuits to defend our civil rights, and we must, along with Julian Assange, cling to our faith that there are still a few sane and rational judges who have not been politically or financially coopted, nor terrorized by the sheer fear of death after a year and half of non-stop propaganda. Those judges will assess the data and side with the truth in defending societies from their bureaucratic tyrants run amok.

13. Conscience and Non-Compliance: The Case of the COVID-19 Vaccine

October 12, 2021
Historic New Castle, Delaware

"How selfish, ignorant, and stupid can people possibly be?!" ask in various ways Emmanuel Macron in France, Jacinda Ardern in New Zealand, Gavin Newsom in California, Bill de Blasio in New York, and even Queen Elizabeth in Britain, along with a surprising number of other public figures, including celebrities, who for some reason have agreed to join in on the global propaganda campaign currently underway. Many political leaders, including U.S. President Joe Biden, Canadian Prime Minister Justin Trudeau, and Victorian (Australia) Premier Daniel Andrews, have repeatedly informed their constituents that they are exasperated by the vaccine hesitancy of their compatriots.

"Do the right thing!" they continue to chant. "Just get the vaccine!" But where carrots and cajoling have failed, governments are now taking up sticks and threats, mandating vaccination for large classes of persons based not on their health profiles — as ethical medical practice would require — but only on where they happen to work or to live.

In truth, there are plenty of epistemologically respectable reasons, firmly grounded in data, for declining to roll up one's sleeve for the COVID-19 "vaccine." Among people who read books, some are wary of Pfizer's track record. The drug giant holds the dubious distinction of paying out the largest fine for healthcare fraud in history.[122] For fifteen years, Pfizer's anti-smoking drug Chantix (varenicline), having received a "priority FDA review," reaped billions of dollars in profits. More than 500 suicides were reportedly committed, and another 2,000 or so attempted, by persons taking the drug. The "suicidal ideation" side effect began to be reported within the first year of the 2006 marketing launch. Chantix was finally pulled from the market in September 2021, not for its untoward psychological effects,[123] but because it had been determined to be carcinogenic.[124]

Johnson & Johnson, too, has a checkered past, having repeatedly lied to consumers about its products, including its widely used baby powder,[125] for decades. AstraZeneca, whose vaccine remained the primary choice in Britain throughout 2021, despite having earned the sobriquet "clot shot" (and having been banned altogether by Denmark[126]), has also been subject to hefty fines for malfeasance, including the off-label marketing of Seroquel (quetiapine).[127] Seroquel has been linked to suicides and other deaths among soldiers to whom the antipsychotic drug was prescribed as a sleep aid.[128] Like the other manufacturers of psychotropic drugs, AstraZeneca has based its marketing claims on short-term, not long-term, studies of its products. Clinical trials in recent years have concluded that placebos are in fact at least as effective as the psychiatric products being peddled to everyone for anything, and less harmful in the long term.[129] As for DARPA-funded Moderna,[130] there are no "skeletons in the closet," because the COVID-19 mRNA therapy is the first Moderna product ever to make it to market.

Even setting aside concerns with the pharmaceutical and biotech firms making a killing from the COVID-19 pandemic, there are specific reasons for doubting the wisdom of undergoing inoculation in this particular case. Most obviously, the elixir being shot into billions of arms all over the world is a treatment touted primarily for its efficacy in averting severe symptoms and death. If one is vulnerable to those effects, then one has some reason for considering the treatment. In fact, according to data readily available from many sources, including the CDC, the vast majority of people are not vulnerable to such effects, so the rational choice of whether to get the jab can only be a matter of personal risk assessment, just as is the choice of whether to undergo any optional medical treatment. Yes, there is a small chance that a healthy person under the age of seventy with no comorbidities will succumb to the virus, develop severe symptoms, require hospitalization, and perhaps even die. But there is also a chance, if ever-so slim, that the person may find himself on the losing end of the adverse effects bell curve, suffering one among dozens of possible complications, including myocarditis, Bell's Palsy, or even death.

The insidious charge of "selfishness" directed toward those who decline the treatment is based upon the old definition of *vaccine* and the idea that the good of society requires everyone to pitch in and do their part for public health. Before the Coronapocalypse, *vaccines* were defined and designed as substances which would prevent transmission of and infection by a disease. If you already had and survived the disease, then you did not need the vaccine, because vaccines were developed specifically to mimic the wondrous workings of the human immune system. The vaccines of the past introduced a small dose of the enemy virus — whether dead or alive — into the body to provoke an immune response so that, should the full force of the wild virus be encountered in the future, the body would already have the needed antibody and T-cell apparatus in place, ready to attack and eliminate the invader rather than allow it to take over and possibly kill its host.

Not only has the concept of *vaccine* been redefined by public health officials so as to subsume the current injections, which do not prevent transmission and infection, but people who have already recovered from COVID-19 are being told that they, too, should undergo vaccination. This is a medically — and indeed logically — dubious prescription, given that the vaccines provoke the body to produce a small subset of the virus (the spike protein), which was already defeated by the previously infected person's body, in the case of anyone who survived. Moreover, numerous studies have demonstrated the robustness of protection acquired through previous infection.[131]

It is no longer a matter of dispute that undergoing inoculation with foreign mRNA to induce one's body to produce a viral spike protein which will jolt the immune system into generating antibodies does not prevent transmission of or infection by COVID-19. Accordingly, this now-debunked early marketing point should not figure into anyone's personal decision at all. We know that cases have continued to spike to new levels exceeding those of a year ago, back when nobody was vaccinated. The accuracy of the testing regimen has been called into question over and over again, but because the same PCR tests used this year were used last year, only time will tell how the tallies will change once the FDA's Emergency Use Authorization of the test expires at the end of 2021.

We also know from the rich body of statistics available from Israel, the most highly vaccinated country on the planet, that what we are witnessing is not, as the propaganda puppets continue to claim, "a pandemic of the unvaccinated." We know that vaccine efficacy wanes rapidly (particularly for the Pfizer product), with a vulnerable vaccinated person's protection dropping from 88% to 47% and continuing to diminish further over time. Many "fully vaccinated" people have been hospitalized and died. So what are we to conclude?

Tellingly, elderly persons and those who for other reasons are more vulnerable to COVID-19 are the only ones in the United States being offered "booster shots" after six months, to elevate their protection to the initial level, which is not 95%, as the marketers initially claimed, but at most 88%, for the most vulnerable persons. Recent studies have revealed that the adverse effects odds are actually worse than the virus odds for some cohorts, including males from the ages of twelve to fifteen, who suffer a greater incidence of myocarditis than other groups after vaccination, making the jab nothing short of irrational for them.[132] We can further deduce from the fact that "boosters" are only being provided to the most vulnerable persons in the United States that invulnerable persons (such as children and healthy adults) never really needed the mRNA treatment in the first place. For anyone who remains confounded by this perhaps astonishing implication, let us spell it out explicitly: if you were "fully vaccinated" many months ago, at some point you will no longer be vaccinated at all. *But the government is not offering you a booster shot?* That's because you number among the vast majority of people who are not vulnerable to COVID-19.

That's right: you, Gentle Double-Jabbed Reader, served as a voluntary subject (*pro bono!*) in an experimental pharmaceutical trial for a product of which you had no need. Instead of being incensed with people who did not roll up their sleeves, you should be angry with the powers that be who persuaded you to undergo an unnecessary medical treatment. And you should be relieved that you were not one of its victims. See the CDC's own Vaccine Adverse Effect Reporting System (VAERS) for more information on that.[133]

Government bureaucrats lie all of the time, Anthony Fauci being only one of the most brazen figures in recent history to claim that his serial prevarication is somehow "noble." Rarely have so many people so openly embraced so many lies. Through a relentless propaganda campaign, a large swath of the population has been persuaded to believe that their neighbors are selfish and even evil for their rational disagreement on a matter of medical choice. Preposterously, in cities such as Los Angeles and New York, proof of vaccination is being demanded for participation in most social activities, despite the fact that booster shots are not currently being offered to healthy young people vaccinated more than six months ago, and previous infection provides robust protection. In other words, the "vaccine passports" being required in such places serve no public health purpose whatsoever but instead constitute a badge of compliance, and are part of a frightening global effort to forge a two-tiered society where "some people are more equal than others."

The extreme, Manichean polarization we are witnessing has been no mean feat of propaganda, rivaled in history only by calls for war in violation of international law, such as the 2003 invasion of Iraq. Some of the people being threatened with the termination of their jobs for refusing to undergo COVID-19 "vaccination" do not have the luxury of living off their savings as an alternative to working. Some among them are heads of households with children to feed. They are facing a moral dilemma: whether to sacrifice the well-being of their family in order to heed their own conscience. For it is indeed a matter of conscience; it is not a matter of need. People have been offered free vaccines for more than nine months in the United States. Some among them chose to decline, for reasons outlined above, or for religious reasons, or for whatever their reasons happened to be. It does not even matter what their reasons were, for human beings have the dignity of choosing what to put into their own bodies.

We should be concerned not only with the disastrous financial consequences for the thousands of people who are now losing their jobs, but also with the moral consequences for a society of persons being coerced to violate their own conscience and renounce their medical freedom. In fact, much more is at stake here than people's livelihood and physical health. We are witnessing a culling of conscience across all sectors of society as individuals who dare to disagree are disparaged, denounced, and marginalized as miscreants whose civil liberties may be taken away, as though they were convicted felons.

The sinister nature of what is unfolding before our very eyes in real time is betrayed in part by the fact that citizens are being ordered to submit to vaccination despite the immunity from legal prosecution of the product companies in the event of negative or even deadly side effects. (This is because of the PREP [Public Readiness and Emergency Preparedness] Act.[134]) If the populace agrees to this pharmaceutical takeover of their very own bodies, then they will no longer have any rights, not even the right to life. They will have become, in effect, slaves. Any pharma goo deemed necessary by the powers that be in the future will, following this precedent, become a condition on the exercise of what were formerly considered citizens' God-given rights to conduct themselves as they please, within the limits of the law. The hitch here is that the laws are being rewritten so as to criminalize medical choice, in a stunning denial of human rights which, lest we forget, resulted only from centuries of hard-fought battles against tyranny, now rearing its ugly head all over again.

Standing up for what is right is never easy in the face of angry mobs fueled by fear. But holding the line is indeed what we must now do. Whatever our personal medical choice happens to be, we should support the healthcare workers who lost their jobs, the dissenting doctors who bravely speak out, and all of the people who have attempted to abide by their conscience in these difficult times. We must defend the perimeters of our own bodies and reject the obnoxious idea that anyone else should be able to decree that we be injected with whatever they happen to believe we should be forced to accept. This is a very slippery slope on which we must refuse to step. If we surrender our bodily autonomy to the government, then we will have nothing left. Wrong is wrong. Do not comply.

14. The Frances Haugen Insurgency

November 8, 2021
Kennewick, Washington

Former Facebook employee Frances Haugen has taken the world by storm by stealing and sharing reams of company communications in which the social media giant's cavalier attitudes toward a range of behaviors among its users are revealed. She compares what she regards as "the Facebook problem" with earlier corporate revelations in history which led to legislation regulating tobacco and automobile use, and she emphasizes that children are specifically at risk from the company's policies. The disgruntled former employee also alleges that Facebook products — in particular, Instagram — harm young women by promoting unhealthy and unrealistic body images.

Despite the vagueness and generality of these complaints, Haugen is being hailed as a "whistleblower" by everyone who agrees with her ideological and political perspective, which is as plain as day: textbook neoliberal, big government, pro-Democratic Party. The objective of the Frances Haugen insurgency is equally manifest: to implement formal government censorship of social media platforms, a literal Ministry of Truth, for "the good" of the people who use them.

The fact that Haugen has been granted such an impressive platform and portrayed throughout the mainstream media as some sort of heroine does not imply that she is a "whistleblower" any more than calling the innocent people killed by bombs "collateral damage" somehow exonerates the killers for their completely avoidable acts of homicide. Frances Haugen, whose vast and highly visible media tour has been funded by Pierre Omidyar, is not, let us be perfectly frank, a whistleblower.[135] This is yet another case where language has been redefined to support a particular political program. Just as "assassination" became "targeted killing" and "torture" became "enhanced interrogation techniques" when authorized by the U.S. president, the concept of "whistleblower" has now been rebranded to cover people who speak out in ways approved of by the very people who provide the speaker with a platform for airing grievances with which all "good" people will agree, with the ultimate aim of expanding the orchestrators' own domain of power and control.

In reality, Haugen has "revealed" only that the social media platform founded by Mark Zuckerberg has not been conducting itself in the manner in which Haugen's associates want it to. Spectacularly enough, Haugen alleges that publicly traded Facebook has been run as — wait for it — a profit-driven company. One might immediately dismiss such a complaint as a failure on the part of the so-called whistleblower to understand the nature of business in a capitalist society. But Haugen holds an M.B.A. from Harvard University. Presumably in securing that credential she was taught that publicly traded companies work for their shareholders and aim to maximize profit. That's what they do. Sure, there are plenty of "woke" companies, which launch "socially conscious" initiatives, but those activities are part and parcel of the marketing apparatus. Erecting a "woke" façade apparently improves the image of a company and thereby increases the sales of its products — at least to the woke. I am not intending here to express cynicism but to state the uncontroversial fact that publicly traded companies which do not keep their shareholders happy eventually fail. Should "wokeness" cut into profits — by alienating self-styled "anti-woke" or "based" customers — then it is bound to be curtailed, at least in the case of any competently run company.

The fact that Haugen has secured such a wide-ranging audience is all the more remarkable given that nearly everyone already knew that Facebook was a profit-driven company. That is precisely why when one creates an auxiliary page at the platform, to promote a book or a small business or product, virtually nobody who likes or follows the page is ever alerted to new content posted there, unless the page owner forks over some funds. The page feature is no doubt a huge moneymaker for the company, as many users feel that it is worth putting Facebook on credit card autopay to ensure that someone — anyone — will see what they have to sell, or to show and to tell.

Ms. Haugen, who touts her own personal risk as evidence of her sincerity, may have stolen documents from Facebook and violated her NDA (non-disclosure agreement), but she has not uncovered any litigable crimes. That's because private businesses have the right to run their companies and, in this case, moderate their content as they please. We know that the Big Tech social media giants censor posts and exclude people who post what they identify as "disinformation" or "hate speech." Up until now, this has been regarded by many liberty advocates as perfectly acceptable, on the grounds that private companies have every right to remove content which they themselves find objectionable or to banish users who violate their terms of service. In their backyard, people must play by their rules. Now, however, the issue has become a test of the First Amendment to the U.S. Constitution, which states:

> Congress shall make no law respecting an establishment of religion, or prohibiting the free exercise thereof; or abridging the freedom of speech, or of the press; or the right of the people peaceably to assemble, and to petition the Government for a redress of grievances.

This provision limits not private businesses but only the government. Indeed, it is specifically designed to protect the people from the government, not the government from the people. Anyone who labels Haugen a "whistleblower" has succumbed to an incredible con job, whereby the First Amendment is to be entirely negated by creating a government-run regulatory body whose role will be to censor content directly, not indirectly, as has been done until now. The reason for this initiative is not that Facebook has acted criminally in maximizing profit, but that they have not been subservient enough to government pressure already put on them to prohibit certain types of content.

Facebook is a profit-driven company, not a branch of the U.S. government. The algorithms used by Facebook do not allow people to see new content organically and chronologically as it is posted by those whom they follow. Instead, Facebook leads users to certain content and prevents them from seeing other content. None of this is done with the intention of promoting extremism. It just happens to be the best way to maximize profit. Haugen's complaints and moralizing are made from a specific TDS (Trump Derangement Syndrome) perspective, the same one which fueled three years of the nugatory Russiagate hunt to prove that Trump was elected only thanks to Vladimir Putin. That the platform has been used by human traffickers is merely a pretext by which to persuade people to believe that it needs to be controlled by a central government authority or Ministry of Truth. In fact, the same argument, *mutatis mutandis*, would apply to the use of vehicles to transport victims. Or to cellphone usage, given that criminals also communicate using those devices.

There are plenty of obvious responses to Haugen's many complaints. Children's use of the Internet, as of the television, should be monitored by their parents, who are responsible for them until they achieve adulthood. Furthermore, seeing pictures and reading texts does not cause cancer and lung disease, and therefore is nothing like smoking cigarettes. Again, where was Frances Haugen (now thirty-seven years old) before the Internet?

Apparently not looking at magazines such as *Vogue*, which have promoted images of extremely thin women for more than a century. Each of her many complaints is similarly simple to defuse, evincing a general conflation of cultural causes and effects.

Yet the story just keeps getting better and better. At the Lisbon Tech Fair on November 1, 2021, Haugen, the keynote speaker, went even so far as to call for the resignation of Facebook CEO Mark Zuckerberg.[136] She claimed that leaving Zuckerberg in place would be a grave error because she believes that 10 million lives are at stake. (What?!) If such a projection does not sound sensationalist to you, then I'd venture to guess that you number among the people who believe that the protest on January 6, 2021, was the worst thing to happen to the United States since the Civil War. And, yes, Haugen has indeed included among her many grievances Facebook's "dangerous" contribution to that nugatory "insurrection" attempt, just in case there were any lingering doubts as to her ideological sympathies.

Haugen is so confident in her self-righteousness (or is it just her security detail?) and so little afraid of Facebook, whose documents she stole, that she seems to believe that she should be able to select the company's CEO. This preposterous conceit should sound familiar, for it is not at all unlike the U.S. government's longstanding practice of decreeing who should govern foreign countries. The sort of CEO favored by Haugen & Co. would be the corporate analogue to Juan Guaidó, whom the U.S. government "recognized" as the true president of Venezuela in 2019, notwithstanding the democratic election of Nicolás Maduro by the people of Venezuela.

The farcical nature of Haugen's obviously scripted, theatrical production is best illuminated by contrast to cases in the real world (not Haugen & Co.'s imagination) where millions of lives are in fact directly at stake — specifically, in the wars of choice continually waged by the United States. The true whistleblowers, who reveal the criminality of what the government is doing and has done, invariably wind up either dead, exiled, or imprisoned under conditions even worse than those of terrorist suspects. Why should that be the case? Because the government wishes not only to prevent these entirely non-violent dissidents from getting the word out but also to deter other possible future whistleblowers from following in their footsteps. Thanks to genuine whistleblower Edward Snowden, we know that the NSA sweeps up all of our cellphone data, regardless of whether or not we have been convicted or are suspected of crimes. Snowden was stripped of his U.S. passport and now resides in Russia.

The persecution of Julian Assange is another case in point. The U.S. government is not pursuing anything approaching justice in this case, for Assange published top secret documents provided to him by whistleblower Bradley (now Chelsea) Manning, among others. Assange, being an Australian national, certainly has no obligation to support the U.S. government and cannot with legal or linguistic propriety be termed a *traitor*. The relentless pursuit of Assange is clearly intended to prevent him from having any further effect on the world. By founding WikiLeaks and revealing what goes on behind the scenes of so-called just wars, Assange had the potential to effect a veritable antiwar revolution. Instead, he is wasting away in prison while his lawyers attempt to prevent his extradition to the United States to face charges of espionage. This despite well-documented criminal violations on the part of the plaintiff, ranging from spying on Assange and his lawyers to plotting to kill him.

The reason why investigative journalists break stories based on stolen documents is that they have discovered news about which the populace is ignorant. WikiLeaks published the "Collateral Murder" video stolen by Private Manning not to glorify Julian Assange but because it showed U.S. soldiers killing Reuters journalists from a helicopter. This was shocking in and of itself, but the accompanying audio recording also revealed the attitudes of the killers toward their victims, including their desire to kill even wounded persons. This was surely news to most people of the United States, and around the world, and it needed to be reported because, in a free society, citizens must know what they are paying for when they file taxes each year. Otherwise, they are being coerced through deception.

Similarly, drone program whistleblowers have sought to alleviate their profound sense of guilt and shame by documenting the horrifying truth for all Americans to see, in the hope that, if only they knew that they were accomplices to murder, then at least some among them would withdraw their support from the serial military interventions in the Middle East. The Obama administration rebranded assassination as "targeted killing" and used that label as their cover for executing, on the basis of purely circumstantial evidence, thousands of persons suspected of collaboration with terrorist groups, in places where there were no U.S. citizens on the ground to protect. We were recently afforded the opportunity to glimpse the "rigor" with which targets were selected by those running the U.S. government's drone program when Zemari Ahmadi, an aid worker, and his entire family were taken out by a Reaper drone in Kabul, Afghanistan, on August 29, 2021.[137]

Anyone who has been listening to the critics and whistleblowers who abandoned the drone program, such as Brandon Bryant,[138] Cian Westmoreland, Stephen Lewis, Michael Haas, and Daniel Hale,[139] already knew that such executions of suspects on the basis of scant evidence have been carried out for years. Of those who have spoken out, Daniel Hale deserves special mention,[140] for he also stole and shared a trove of documents, published online as *The Drone Papers*,[141] and later in book form as *The Assassination Complex* (2017),[142] which revealed to the public precisely what was graphically displayed in the strike carried out on August 29, 2021. Persons "outside areas of active hostility" are targeted based on cellphone SIM card data, the claims of bribed informants looking to procure wads of cash, and drone footage appearing to confirm the killers' prior beliefs that the suspects are indeed terrorists. None of the victims were ever provided with the opportunity to demonstrate their innocence before being incinerated, and none have been permitted to surrender — most having had no idea that they were about to be erased from existence by a missile launched from a drone. In other words, this practice of "targeted killing" blatantly violates the Geneva Conventions prohibiting the summary execution of unarmed soldiers and the requirement of taking as prisoners any of those who agree to lay down their arms.

Where is Daniel Hale today? He certainly was not invited to speak before the U.S. Congress or as a special guest before the British Parliament about the malfeasance of the U.S. and U.K. governments in executing innocent human beings on the basis of shoddy evidence. Instead, Hale, a genuine whistleblower, who committed a crime in order to reveal the much worse crimes of his government, is now serving a nearly four-year sentence (forty-five months) in federal prison for sharing with the public the truth about the drone program. Despite the gravity of Hale's revelations, no one in the mainstream media discussed the outrageousness of killing suspects after having offered them no opportunity to demonstrate their innocence, nor even to surrender, before carbonizing them in places where no U.S. citizen's life was at stake. Instead, Daniel Hale was hardly mentioned by anyone in the mainstream media at all. Upon his conviction, a line or two to the effect that another former soldier had been convicted under the Espionage Act could be found in a few media outlets. *Oh well, another spy bites the dust!*

Given the obvious role of the mainstream media in supporting the War Party duopoly, having persuaded the populace to believe that "offensive military action is defensive," "suspects are terrorists," and "we are good, and they are evil," perhaps the Frances Haugen insurgency was bound to happen eventually. Here we are, in 2021, in a world where political operatives speak out not to reveal crimes committed by the government but to strengthen its power to suppress dissent through undermining the First Amendment to the U.S. Constitution, thereby permitting the commission of even more crimes by the state.

Make no mistake: Haugen's repeated expression of concern for children is a rhetorical tactic to garner support for the federal government's usurpation of the power of private companies to determine what may and may not be said and shown on their platforms. Just as the claim that infants were being ripped from incubators by Saddam Hussein's henchmen in Kuwait was instrumental in galvanizing support for the ill-begotten First Gulf War on Iraq in 1991, Haugen makes a big show of caring about the children supposedly harmed by Facebook in order to persuade Congress to establish a broad regulatory power not currently enjoyed by the government.

The potential for misuse of this open-ended expansion of executive power is well illustrated by the 2002 AUMF (Authorization for Use of Military Force). Recall that in October 2002, the U.S. Congress ratified the AUMF on the grounds that President George W. Bush needed to protect the world from Iraq's dictator, who was said to possess WMD (weapons of mass destruction) and the intention to share them with factional terrorists. In the subsequent two decades, the AUMF was wielded repeatedly as the alleged authorization for every president to kill anyone anywhere he wanted to, even "outside areas of active hostility."

For now, words still have meanings, and 2 + 2 = 4. But the very real danger to the citizens of a republic inherent to Haugen's initiative cannot be exaggerated. The establishment of a full-fledged Ministry of Truth would stifle, if not altogether eliminate, dissent. For such a regulatory apparatus would possess the means to prevent its own dismantlement for generations to come, by silencing all who disagree with the government, denouncing them as purveyors of disinformation or, worse, traitors.

Needless to say, in the current vexed climate of COVID hysteria, the potential for further usurpation of civil liberties is very real. If the government secures the means to control exclusively what is allowed to be reported as "The Science," and uses that power to impose broad new restrictions and requirements upon citizens, up to and including the need to inject whatever pharmaceutical product has been touted as the latest panacea by profit-driven companies, then the formerly free inhabitants of a republic will have been rendered into the slaves of a tyrannical state.

Given the outrageousness of Haugen's call for Zuckerberg's resignation, one hopes that people will come to question her motives and think through the broader implications of her demands. Perhaps the most beneficial outcome of the Frances Haugen insurgency will be to permit us to determine, by their reactions to Haugen, who among the current crop of politicians are in fact closet totalitarians, their rhetoric about the importance of democracy notwithstanding.

When is a whistleblower not a whistleblower? When she's a politically driven hack who promotes censorship in order to expand the power of the government by diminishing the power of citizens to express themselves.

15. The Gaslighting Government

December 6, 2021
Joseph, Oregon

The film *Gaslight* (1944), directed by George Cukor and starring Ingrid Bergman and Charles Boyer, relays the story of a con artist, Sergis Bauer, who under the assumed name of Gregory Anton seduces and marries a young woman, Paula Alquist. The smitten bride has no idea that her charming husband murdered her aunt, Alice Alquist, who left behind a home in London where a cache of priceless jewels is stashed somewhere in the attic. The newlyweds move into the home, which Paula has inherited, and the husband proceeds to dig through the contents of the attic in an impassioned effort to locate the jewels. In order to accomplish this aim, he must keep his wife inside the house while he goes out at night, ostensibly to work in his studio. Instead, he accesses the attic of the house from an alley entrance.

While rummaging around upstairs, directly above his wife's head, Bauer makes noises, and his use of a lamp causes the gaslight downstairs to flicker, naturally raising questions in his wife's mind. He quells her concerns about what is going on by persuading her to believe that her perceptions are mere figments of her imagination and indeed evidence that she is going mad. To bolster this claim, he takes down paintings and hides them, after which he insists that she was the one to have moved them, despite having no memory of having done so. The criminal comes very close to having his wife committed to an insane asylum, at which point he would be free to search the entire house without raising any suspicions whatsoever, because she would be out of the picture. Just in the nick of time, the scheme is thwarted by the arrival on the scene of a hero (played by Joseph Cotten) to save the day.

The term *gaslighting* has come to refer thus to the phenomenon by which people are systematically persuaded to question their own perceptions of reality. It is a tactic deployed by sociopaths and psychological abusers who persuade docile people to accept whatever they say, no matter how preposterous, and no matter how much it conflicts with the deliverances of their very own senses. Such psychological manipulators are greatly aided in this endeavor through their persuasion of other people to agree with their version of what is going on.

Governments which exert influence over the mainstream media are quite adept at this sort of manipulation, as is well illustrated by the buildup to every war. Those who oppose bombing campaigns are portrayed as cowards and traitors, if not miscreants, by war profiteers who manage to persuade much of the populace of the necessity of military intervention, despite the fact that it will kill innocent civilians who have nothing whatsoever to do with the behavior of the leaders said to necessitate recourse to war. Gross injustices are in this way portrayed as not only permissible and just, but also obligatory.[143]

The gaslighting tactic was equally well illustrated by the U.S. government's response to the revelation that illegal mass surveillance had been undertaken against the entire population. Rather than expressing compunction for the crimes committed, those responsible instead insisted that no one was really looking at any of the data anyway. This line was further bolstered by cries throughout the media that "Innocent people have nothing to hide!" The scandal was shortly thereafter forgotten by much of the populace whose right to privacy had been violated by their very own government.

Similarly, when WikiLeaks published the "Collateral Murder" video depicting civilians, including Reuters journalists, executed point blank from an Apache helicopter by the U.S. military, people all over the world were appalled. The powers that be responded to the public uproar by vowing to investigate. But they ultimately concluded that no crime had been committed, for the soldiers had acted in accordance with their rules of engagement. In other words, if you thought that you were witnessing with your very own eyes the unthinkable murder of civilians on film, you were wrong, according to the gaslighting government. Likewise, when the U.S. government defined *dead suspects* as *dead terrorists*, by labeling them *Enemy Killed in Action* (EKIA), even when located outside areas of active hostilities, they effectively decreed that they could use lethal drones to kill anyone anywhere for any reason.[144] Having been told by the gaslighting government that everything done in their name was intended to keep them safe, the populace generally acquiesced to this usurpation even of citizens' rights to a fair trial before being summarily executed at the caprice of bureaucrats.

Predictably enough, given the precedents already set by the U.S. government, when ten civilians were killed by a Reaper drone in Kabul, Afghanistan, on August 29, 2021,[145] the Pentagon concluded their investigation of the case by claiming that they had committed no crimes in destroying those people, seven of whom were children. But that was only because the killers had not violated the laws of war rewritten by none other than themselves and, again, according to which anyone can be eliminated at any time for any reason, provided only that the government has determined that this should be done.

These examples underscore the fact that political power once captured is rarely ceded and progressively expands in the absence of resistance, a principle equally well illustrated by the handling of the COVID-19 crisis by governments the world over. Entire populations have been kept in a continuous state of uncertainty, never knowing what they will be forbidden from doing next. Vaccine passports, following the trajectory of circular stickers on floors, have swept through the First World, having been taken up in Israel, Canada, and throughout Europe, in addition to cities such as New York and Los Angeles, with millions of citizens now denied the right to socialize, use public transportation, go shopping, work, drive, or lead any semblance of a normal life without first presenting their health credentials. In Australia, healthy people in the Northern Territory who have been in contact with persons who tested positive for COVID-19 are being sent to quarantine camps.[146]

Fear and uncertainty are powerful tools by which to gain, retain, and augment government control because everything that officials do is claimed to benefit their constituents. Whether it is the War on Terror or the current health crisis, all bureaucrats everywhere sincerely profess to be doing no more and no less than trying to protect their compatriots' lives. That's the standard refrain, rehearsed each time a new policy or intervention is imposed, or a civil liberty stripped away. There is no need to assess the consequences of well-intended initiatives, because the docile populace charitably permits government officials to plod along with their failed policies, no matter what they do — even when they kill citizens themselves. That was how the fiasco in Afghanistan dragged on for two decades, and that is why even when the *Fool's Errand*[147] was at last recognized for what it was by people in the position to effect change, a number of pundits and politicians protested in response, insisting that pulling out was a mistake.

As in the case of the many liberty-restricting measures adopted throughout the Global War on Terror, the attempt by governments to force their citizenry to subject themselves to serial injections of novel substances into their bodies is said by supporters to be intended only to protect them. All across the globe, arbitrary punishments are being exacted against those who refuse to comply. This despite the ongoing protests by thousands of people for months on end in countries such as France and Australia, where the protesters obviously have not dropped dead from their failure to comply with public health measures, whether masking, vaccination, or social distancing.

The government of Austria recently announced that all of its unvaccinated population would be locked down. Shortly thereafter, the lockdown was extended to cover vaccinated persons as well. It seems likely that this was a part of the gaslighting government's general strategy to demonize the unvaccinated as the cause of the loss of the freedom of the vaccinated, under the assumption that the latter would increase pressure on the former to comply. Ratcheting up their campaign to vaccinate every citizen, the Austrian government has further announced a hefty €7,200 fine to be extracted from those who persist in resisting.[148]

The polarization of people into two antithetical groups, the vaccinated and the so-called anti-vaxxers, has been very effective in shutting down nearly all debate into serious questions regarding the efficacy of COVID-19 public health policies. When case numbers surge, this is immediately blamed upon the unvaccinated, as is the appearance of each new variant, even though a number of virologists maintain that the decision to vaccinate the entire population during a pandemic (rather than waiting some time) itself led to the creation of new variants, as the virus fought to survive in vaccinated hosts by wriggling its way around the spike protein antibodies created in response to the mRNA injections.

Because fully half of the population persists in a state of manifest terror at the prospect of death by virus, the major challenge today for free people has become to defend our shrinking liberties from governments which have clearly been captured by pro-Big Pharma forces. It is stunning that so many people have been persuaded to believe that they should do whatever Pfizer wants them to, despite the company's well-documented history of malfeasance and fraud.[149] Only the climate of fear and uncertainty continuously cultivated by media outlets (sponsored by Pfizer!) and government spokespersons can explain this group behavior phenomenon, which exhibits many characteristics of religious cults. It goes without saying that cult leaders are exemplary gaslighters, for their followers occupy a world of the cult leader's creation. *New Normal*, anyone?

Cults are created and flourish in a climate of fear and/or uncertainty. A self-proclaimed special leader with unique access to The Truth arrives on the scene to offer himself magnanimously to a group of people as the solution to the dire situation. In the United States, gaslighter *par excellence* Dr. Anthony Fauci has become the go-to guru, despite having repeatedly issued contradictory guidance on everything from masks to lockdowns to travel bans to natural immunity to virus origin and the wisdom of mandatory vaccination. When confronted with his contradictions, Fauci has claimed that he lied for the good of the people. In fact, none of this behavior is surprising, because the way in which cult leaders maintain control of their groups is by continually rehydrating the very sense of uncertainty and fear which led people to join in the first place.

One of the most graphic uses of gaslighting by public health officials has been their utter refusal to acknowledge the reality of natural immunity through previous infection. There is no other case of a disease known to humankind and for which a vaccine exists, where previously infected and fully recovered people are exhorted to undergo vaccination. That's because vaccines are specifically designed to provoke a response from the immune system. Vaccines incite the production of antibodies and T-cells which protect a person from the invasion of a virus. If the immune system did not protect infected people, then they would all be dead. Instead, more than 99% of people who contract COVID-19 survive, clearly demonstrating the efficacy of natural immunity. Most significantly, if the human immune system could not hold its own against a virus, then no vaccine designed to jolt the human immune system into fighting that same virus could possibly be effective. It is a case of gaslighting *extraordinaire* to claim that the immune system will only work if one is vaccinated with an elixir whose efficacy depends on the ability of the immune system to work.

A second, and equally remarkable, case of gaslighting occurred in the initial marketing campaign for the mRNA products, when representatives of the product companies exuberantly claimed that the vaccines offered up to 95% efficacy against severe illness and death, which was a protection *already enjoyed naturally* by the vast majority of the population pre-vaccine, because they were never vulnerable to serious illness from the virus in the first place. Having been persuaded to believe in the manifestly preposterous conjunction that natural immunity is worthless, and mRNA "vaccines" reliant for their efficacy on natural immunity are necessary, much of the populace stands ready to accept nearly any other contradiction which comes their way, even when it entails the surrender of their civil liberties.

Leaders continue to spout out absurdities such as "We're going to protect vaccinated workers from unvaccinated coworkers." The gaslighting government has been relentless in its quest to persuade skeptical citizens that their perceptions of what is going on are all wrong.[150] Parents who worry that their children are being harmed by requirements to wear masks, which reduce oxygen flow to their brains and prevent them from learning appropriate behavior through reacting to facial cues, have been told by the gaslighting government (Jen Psaki, Biden's press secretary) that masks are just like "hair ribbons." Those who wonder whether financial interests (such as stock holdings and patent ownership) might possibly influence bureaucrats' policy recommendations are shutdown as "conspiracy theorists." Obviously, there is no merit to the idea that non-vaccine therapies were proscribed for the simple reason that Emergency Use Authorization (EUA) of the experimental vaccines required that there be no alternative therapies available. That's just another conspiracy theory, according to the gaslighting government.

The list of ideas which fly in the face of common sense but are fully embraced by true believers is amazing to behold. Clearly, it makes perfect sense to require healthy people to undergo experimental medical interventions with unknown long-term side effects. There is nothing wrong with requiring healthy people to submit to medical treatments as a condition on their current and future employment, even though the treatment in question does not prevent transmission of or infection by the disease whose symptoms it is designed to moderate. It is perfectly logical to prevent people from traveling from one country to another where the rate of infection is even worse than the country of origin. The government is better situated to determine which medications a patient should ingest than is that patient's own doctor. There is nothing at all alarming about the government sending out the vaccine police to ensure compliance with what public health officials believe should be the treatment of healthy people, despite knowing nothing about their medical history or circumstances. It is perfectly fine to mandate that healthy people undergo experimental injections while protecting the manufacturers from legal repercussions in the event of adverse effects up to and including death. Cloth masks have no prophylactic benefit against viruses whose size is smaller than the pores of the cloth, but people should be required to wear them anyway. Health passports do not prevent infection and transmission, because the "vaccines" which they document do not prevent infection and transmission, but people should nonetheless be required to have them in order to be able to participate in society. It is entirely normal for democratically elected leaders to upbraid their constituents as though they were naughty children and threaten them with punishments when they decline to take drugs of which they have no need.

The list goes on and on, and so long as the (for the most part) scientifically illiterate populace continues to bleat "Listen to The Science!" under the assumption that Dr. Anthony Fauci, a mere man, is the apotheosis of the enormous edifice of all scientific knowledge, then they will continue to accept new and arbitrary policies. The idea that lockdown, quarantine, masking, and vaccination requirements will continue on until COVID-19 disappears from the face of the earth has been successfully insinuated into the minds of the Branch Covidians, even though "the virus" will continue to mutate, just as coronaviruses have always done.

Once lured into a gaslighter's web, it becomes progressively more difficult for people to be debriefed as time goes on. They have invested, made sacrifices, and embraced a narrative which becomes more and more compelling, even in the face of conflicting evidence. Human nature is such that no one wants to admit that he has been fooled. Accordingly, instead of blaming at least some of the millions of deaths of Americans throughout the pandemic on the poor policies with which they themselves complied, the followers of Fauci & Co. remain steadfast in their belief that the death toll would have been much worse had they not agreed to do whatever their local health authorities told them to.

For years, companies in the mRNA therapy business were waiting to test their products on human beings, and with the sudden appearance of COVID-19 their opportunity at last arrived. Advocates of universal vaccination are by now so intransigent in their beliefs that they are not bothered in the least by evidence that males in the age cohort 12–17 years are at greater risk from myocarditis post-vaccination than from the virus itself while unvaccinated.[151] The strident call to inoculate small children with next to no vulnerability to COVID-19 is equally perplexing. Before 2020, few people would have rallied to inject perfectly healthy children with experimental elixirs designed to protect *other* people from a virus to which the children themselves were not vulnerable. It is shocking that parents would offer their children up as guinea pigs in what is manifestly an experimental trial for a product of which they have no need.

Impervious to statistical data which belies the story they have been persuaded to believe — such as the relatively good outcomes in places such as Florida and Sweden, and the poor outcomes in California and New York, in addition to the "inexplicable" success story of largely unvaccinated Africa, where vaccine hesitancy is rife and many non-vaccine remedies have been widely used — the true believers continue to insist that Fauci's decrees must be heeded. This despite the fact that the virus death toll of 2021 was greater than that of 2020, even after widespread uptake of the "vaccine" so vigorously promoted as the solution to the crisis.

Nonetheless, according to the gaslighting government, this is a "pandemic of the unvaccinated," reinforcing in the minds of half the population that every single COVID-19 death is caused directly by the evil "anti-vaxxers" who decline the treatment. In fact, it has become increasingly clear that the virus is untamable and endemic, as data from highly vaccinated Israel and Gibraltar strongly suggest. Ignorant of or impervious to this data, the "good" vaccinated are being told by their gaslighting governments that if they do not present themselves for booster shots at regular intervals (Britain recently shortened the period of eligibility from six to three months[152]), then they, too, will number among the irresponsible, unvaccinated killers.

In the face of crisis, leaders are inclined to follow the simple precept "Do something! Do anything!" — the false assumption being that inaction is always worse than action. Having once implemented new policies, leaders are protected by the inaccessibility of counterfactual outcomes, and they always insist that things would have been much worse had they not done what they did. Educated people, however, are now well aware that the government's Global War on Terror itself led to a groundswell of support for the originally quite small group of extremists known as Al Qaeda, and the creation of factional franchises which spread throughout the Middle East and Africa. Similarly, we know that many of the excess deaths over the course of the past two years were caused not by the COVID-19 virus but by the political policies imposed in response to it.

In some parts of the world, the average age of persons killed by COVID-19 has been greater than the actuary tables would have predicted, had the virus never emerged. In contrast, the rise in suicides and drug overdoses among young people, most of whom were not even vulnerable to COVID-19, is most plausibly explained by the draconian political policies preventing them from living what should have been their carefree lives. Not unrelated to the destruction of thousands of small businesses caused directly by government lockdowns, homelessness has increased dramatically, as any inhabitant of a major U.S. city can attest, with the sobering sight of vast tent encampments filling the sidewalks in front of shuttered stores for blocks on end.

Meanwhile, as was predicted by critics back in 2020, strict lockdown and medical triage policies have had as a further tragic effect that people terrified of contracting what they were propagandized to believe was the Black Death were prevented, not only by their own fear, but also by policies postponing routine screenings, from seeking even necessary medical interventions such as chemotherapy and surgery. In the U.K. alone, an estimated 50,000 early cancer diagnoses were missed.[153] Yet government leaders and their appointees have doubled down on their failed policies, despite all of the evidence that they have been blinded by a monomaniacal obsession with one cause of death to the exclusion of any other of the many problems in society. Disturbingly, some medical facilities now refuse to treat the unvaccinated, even for serious illnesses which may culminate in their deaths.

Dozens of peer-reviewed scientific papers have confirmed the rational grounds for skepticism harbored by "non-compliant" citizens, but the gaslighting government plunders ahead undeterred. For they know that their devotees, having lived since 2020 in a state of profound uncertainty, terrified by what was made to seem the looming specter of their imminent death, will agree to anything, up to and including the usurpation of their bodily autonomy.

If you, Skeptical Citizen, reject The New Normal, then there is evidently something wrong with you. The very last thing which anyone should care about is whether the government itself caused the pandemic by funding the gain-of-function research used to create the COVID-19 virus.

16. Is Virtue Signaling Vicious?

December 27, 2021
Holladay, Utah

Virtue signaling — the practice of highlighting what one takes to be one's own moral superiority, often by loudly denouncing the character and comportment, including the speech, of other people — has become a dominant mode of rhetoric throughout social media and network television. *Virtue theory*, in contrast, is a teleological approach to normative morality concerned with how actions affect one's soul or character. Historians of philosophy usually trace virtue theory to Aristotle's *Nicomachean Ethics*, the first extant articulation of ideas such as that habits build character, and virtues represent "the golden mean" along a continuum of two vicious extremes. Courage, for example, lies between the two extremes of cowardice and recklessness, according to Aristotle.

It seems unlikely that many of the people who engage in virtue signaling have any genuine interest in the state of anybody's soul. Certainly shrieking in outrage is unlikely to change anyone's comportment, much less his beliefs, and yet many people persist in the practice anyway, in part because it is both contagious and addictive. The structure of Twitter, in particular, makes it easy to react in a kneejerk way to short proclamations with which one disagrees. It is in fact very difficult, if not impossible, to carry out reason-based debates in the allotted 280-character spaces of a Tweet. It furthermore requires a degree of discipline to refrain from shrieking back at shrieking trolls on Twitter, even while knowing that many of them may well be bots — or unreasonable facsimiles…

Having visited in 2021 several different U.S. cities, including Boston, Denver, Seattle, Salt Lake City, and Austin, where prominently displayed lawn signs profess the "enlightened" beliefs of the people residing there, I have been puzzling over the strange new phenomenon of essentially advertising one's own "virtue." I presume that what is being asserted is moral rather than epistemological superiority, because most of the proclamations on these signs do not contain much in the way of propositional content. "Love is love" is tautological, but "Black lives matter" and "Science is real" also do not represent any sort of cognitive breakthrough. For that reason, whenever I spot one of these signs, I find myself wondering how many people there are who really do believe the literal antitheses of the statements displayed. It would seem that "Human lives matter" implies that "Black lives matter," so there is a hidden insinuation in these pronouncements: that people who do not overtly profess the slogans on signs do not in fact agree and therefore constitute some sort of affront to good people everywhere. They despicably deny the humanity of black people and the deliverances of the scientific enterprise, among other things.

Yet it has become abundantly clear that the disagreements at issue are not really about the simple statements, *per se*. Instead, the banal expressions appear to be code for far more substantial and controversial positions, such as that "George Floyd was a hero," and "Climate change is the most pressing problem facing us today." In this way, nailing a sign in one's front yard is a performative way of broadcasting that one belongs to the right club, and may explain the preponderance of such signs in some neighborhoods, where a veritable "war of the signs" is underway. (On one street in Somerville, Massachusetts, I saw "Black Lives Matter" and "Blue Lives Matter" placards displayed before adjacent homes.) Anecdotally, I can report that "Black Lives Matter" signs are far more common than "Blue Lives Matter" signs, so it seems that the inhabitants of some left-leaning neighborhoods may feel that by failing to post one of the rainbow signs displaying the beliefs of the inhabitants of the house, they may be taken implicitly to ally themselves with the ideological enemy, deplorable Trump supporters and the like.

Alas, in the age of social media, many people appear to labor under the delusion that it suffices to have a "right-minded" opinion in order to be morally superior. This tendency was dialed up significantly during the Trump years, when the stark reality of what can only be termed *tribalism* became impossible to deny. "You're either with us, or you're against us!" serves politicians well during the buildup to every war, but now it has infected civil society to the point where many people reflexively revile others who disagree with them on either Trump or the COVID-19 shots, facilely concluding that they must be not just idiots but also morally depraved.

Millions of Trump haters appear to believe not only that Trump is worthy of their abject abhorrence, but also that they are superior to Trump supporters, who have somehow failed to recognize the former president's abhorrent character. *Shockingly*, they lament, *millions of poor benighted souls verily celebrate the man as their savior!* These polarized attitudes toward Trump are based on beliefs about what he does and why — about which there is considerable disagreement. Mindless worship of a political leader may be wrongheaded, but is it *vicious?*

To take another example, millions of people have put Dr. Anthony Fauci on a pedestal as their savior from the scourge of COVID-19. Interestingly enough, there seems to be a good deal of overlap between Trump haters and Fauci worshipers, which strongly suggests that the etiology of afflictions such as TDS (Trump Derangement Syndrome) and COVID Hysteria are traceable to CNN, MSNBC, and the like. Indeed, at this point in history, the most reliable determinant of whether any given person hates Trump and adores Fauci would seem to be not his education, social or economic status, or state of residence, but whether he watches television and, if so, whether he spends his time at CNN or Fox News.

Of course, we often arrive at our beliefs through entirely random and arbitrary processes. We may be absolutely convinced that we are right — *Murder is wrong!* — but do we deserve any moral credit for having arrived at such a view? I suspect that it is this confusion which leads some people to despise critics. They mistakenly believe that a critic is asserting moral authority, when in fact he or she is making only an epistemological — or, at the most basic level, a logical — objection to what appears to be a manifest falsehood or contradiction. Calling George W. Bush and Tony Blair "war criminals" is to condemn them, but it is also to assert what the speaker takes to be a fact, for if the 2003 war on Iraq was a violation of international law, then its perpetrators were war criminals, and all of those killed in the conflict were victims, whether directly or indirectly, of premeditated, intentional homicide, better known as *murder*.

Moral rhetoric is intrinsically complicated because we all have limited perspectives, and it would seem that one person's incisive critic is another person's shrieking troll. Being of a naturally critical bent, and inclined to sit down and write when questions pop up in my mind, I can attest that some people do consider just about any form of criticism to be an obnoxious, insolent, and self-indulgent form of "virtue signaling." They may appreciate intelligence in an abstract way, but when it comes after their cherished beliefs, that's a completely different story. Witness the plight of Socrates, the case of Julian Assange, or any of the countless other, unnamed dissidents destroyed by their governments over the course of history.

How dare you suggest that there may be weaknesses and contradictions in my views! Who are you *to find fault with* my *opinions and beliefs?* These sorts of reactions —

typically angry — to attempts to highlight problems with fervently held dogmas have led me to reflect upon whether there is any significant distinction to be drawn between, say, screaming that someone is selfish for declining a "vaccine" which is purported not to stop transmission and infection but to moderate symptoms, and pointing out that voluntary obesity has contributed to hospital resource shortages throughout the Coronapocalypse because an estimated 78% of the people who die of COVID-19 are in fact obese.

At the same time that name-calling has become the rule rather than the exception in responding to anyone who happens to disagree — not only on social media, but also throughout the propagandized mainstream outlets which were formerly homes to journalism — one also occasionally encounters gentle exhortations to "Be Kind." Only this morning, during a brisk walk on this cold and crisp winter day in Utah, I spotted an SUV with a license plate reading "B Kind." (I immediately inferred that "Be Kind" had already been nabbed by another, even more enlightened thinker.) Even more so than the yard signs, the exhortation to "Be Kind" may in fact embody a contradiction of sorts, suggesting, as it seems to, that those who see the license plate are going to be mean unless they are told to do the opposite. The form of speech is an imperative, an order, a command. But is it really "kind" to order people around, or to suggest that, left to their own devices, they would naturally be mean?

The "Be Kind" trend may have been popularized in part by talk show host Ellen DeGeneres, around the time when she was explaining her friendship with war criminal George W. Bush. (Oh, was that *mean*?) I would be surprised if very many people believed that kindness is somehow wrong, and, in general, all other things being equal, being kind does seem to be a good thing to do. But my distinct impression from the sometimes hostile reactions to my own critical writings is that some people believe that the very act of criticism is itself mean — or even cruel. Is it "mean" to point out the manifest inconsistencies embraced by other people? Perhaps in some circumstances it can be. But critics such as myself do this a lot. To stop calling out contradictions would require some of us to stop talking altogether. Perhaps we have a "Socrates complex," but, for better or worse, that is who we are.

One way of resolving this problem is to distinguish between insulting people and arguing with them. *Ad hominem* "arguments" are fallacious because they are only insults masquerading as criticism. Telling a person that he is stupid or ugly, *tout court*, is quite different from saying that he holds contradictory views or supports a war which will kill thousands of innocent people, even while claiming to believe that it is wrong to kill innocent people. If "kindness" requires us to remain silent when the government sends troops abroad to deploy homicidal weapons against unarmed, non-threatening persons, then perhaps the world would be better off with less "kindness" and a bit more "mean" but honest critical thinking.

Again, is there a difference between denouncing someone as a "fascist" and exposing the lies and hypocrisy of governments which claim to champion human rights while running perpetual motion bombing campaigns, leaving "collateral damage" victims everywhere in their wake? I have found myself indulging in a bit of the former of late, ever since the president of France, Emmanuel Macron, announced his intention to punish the entire population of unvaccinated inhabitants of his land, rendering them outcasts from the society in which they live, prohibited from mingling with compliant (= "good") people in cafes, bars, restaurants, clubs, and shopping malls, all for the "crime" of having refused to volunteer in an experimental drug trial. Handing out carrots was fine for a while — until it turned out that many citizens found them not enticing in the least, at which point some European governments, even that of Germany, whose earlier abysmal behavior led to the drafting of the Nuremberg Code (see Appendix B), resorted to picking up big sticks.

Taken out of context, an outburst such as *"Macron Fasciste!"* could be regarded as a case of virtue signaling, for it would seem to imply that the speaker, in contrast to Macron, is not a fascist. As I virtually emote *"Macron Fasciste!"* however, my interpretation of what he is doing also embodies a criticism of his violation of French people's rights, which I must figure out a way to explain to those who do not themselves recognize what is problematic about it, lest my words fall on deaf ears. It is easier said than done to persuade others to listen to a rival position with an open mind, and the responses of those whose beliefs are challenged by critics is often emotional, not rational, as is nowhere better illustrated than in the midst of the COVID-19 crisis, during which a frightening degree of certainty has impelled the "Listen to The Science!" crowd to lash out hysterically at anyone who disagrees. It does not seem to matter in the least how seemingly intransigent beliefs were formed. Anyone who dares to adduce new studies or evidence which conflict with the March 2020 CNN/BBC narrative is immediately denounced all over social media and on many networks for spouting "disinformation," as though the television were somehow the sole and authoritative source of The Truth.

The "Listen to The Science!" crowd appears to be signaling what they take to be their own epistemological humility in deferring unerringly to "the experts," even though the ones who regularly appear on television often have financial interests in promoting the Big Pharma line. Indeed, some of the news shows unabashedly showcase Pfizer as a sponsor. The millions of people apparently prepared to hook up to an IV drip of "boosters" for the remainder of their lives, far from being virtuous, strike me as both frightened and confused, which explains why they respond with such vehemence to anyone who points out even scientifically respectable grounds for skepticism. But because individuals themselves bear the brunt of their own decisions, and indeed become who they are through choosing to act in the ways in which they do, they are entitled to disagree on risk-benefit analyses. As with all other decisions, the choice of which medical treatments to undergo is a highly personal one.

Given the entirely unsystematic means through which we arrive at our beliefs, it seems likely that each of us holds at least some contradictory views, which is precisely why we can engage endlessly in heated debates over every matter under the sun. We all change some of our views over the course of our life — though not all at the same time. It would be irrational not to modify beliefs in the light of new revelations, and as the COVID-19 story continues to unfurl in real time, rational people stand ready to acknowledge when they were wrong. The purpose of rational debate is not to prove that we are right but to figure out which beliefs should be abandoned in the face of evidence and logic.

The proper end of debate is not the glorification of whoever "wins" the argument but the ascertainment of the truth or, at the very least, the elimination from contention of a false or misguided belief. Censorship makes this impossible to do, assuming as it does that The Truth has already been ascertained, and all expressions of disagreement, no matter their source or intention, must be stopped. Tactically speaking, the suppression of the speech of those who hold what the censors take to be offensive opinions seems unlikely to change anyone's view and may well exacerbate divisions among those who disagree. But there is a far more fundamental problem with censorship. Like it or not, virtue signaling, and emotive outbursts more generally, are expressed through language, the very tool essential to rational discourse. Whether a statement or exclamation strikes us as puzzling, amusing, repulsive, hateful, or even vicious, we must tolerate it and resist all calls to censorship. “Selective free speech” is a contradiction in terms.

17. The Pharma Revolution Is Being Televised

February 1, 2022
Holladay, Utah

Marketing is essentially the art of persuading people to buy what they would not have bought, left to their own devices. This is achieved through manipulating either desires or perceptions of need. People who do not watch television are exposed to much less advertising of consumer products than are people who do. Similarly, the less time one spends surfing the Internet, expressing either explicit or implicit interest in buying possible products, the fewer items there will likely be in one's various shopping carts, not only because marketers now target people with ads catering to their preferences, but also because one will be exposed to fewer advertisements overall. Big corporations have enormous marketing budgets because advertising works: people often buy what they have been persuaded to believe that they should buy, choosing products with familiar names or whose alleged virtues have been extolled to them through one means or another.

The conspicuous consumption induced by mass-market advertising campaigns may or may not be a vice, but it would be difficult to deny that people do not believe themselves to need a product which they do not know to exist. Correlatively, if they do not believe themselves to suffer from a particular disease, then they will not typically seek out a medical treatment for it. Before 1997, direct-to-consumer advertising of pharmaceutical products was prohibited in the United States, as it is still today throughout most of the world. The presumption against the direct promotion of drugs to patients themselves is grounded in the concern that untutored persons might be persuaded, purely on the basis of seductive advertisements, to pursue treatments of which they have no need.

Throughout history it has been regarded as the role of doctors to recommend possible courses of treatment to patients who require medical intervention. Modern pharmaceutical companies naturally vie for the attention of doctors, in the hopes that they will choose their products over those of competitors. Physicians are the primary readers of journals and magazines featuring articles relaying the results of clinical trials interwoven with advertisements summarizing the virtues of newly manufactured drugs, along with others still under patent. Since 1997, however, patients themselves have been targeted by drug ads as well, through not only television and radio broadcasts but also the Internet. The marketing logic which governs new products in general governs pharmaceutical products in particular.

One must first be informed that a disease exists before attempting to ascertain whether one exhibits its symptoms and should undergo a course of palliative treatment. Healthy people do not usually spend their time fretting over diseases, and throughout most of the twentieth century, people who spent their days poring over medical encyclopedias in order to determine what ailments they might possibly suffer from were widely regarded as *hypochondriacs*, who used medical pretexts to seek out attention and treatment when in fact there was nothing physically wrong with them. Likewise, most parents do not pore over reference books to identify diseases ascribable to their ostensibly healthy children. When the FDA (under the influence of the pharmaceutical industry) lifted the ban on direct-to-consumer advertising of medical products, everything changed, as patients began to request from their doctors pills which they had learned about through commercials specifically designed by marketing departments to maximize sales.

The medical interventions which a doctor is inclined to recommend have always been determined in part by reigning scientific beliefs regarding which diseases exist and can be eliminated or alleviated. Medical conditions, however, are partitioned and diseases delineated by conventions which transform over time. What were for many years deemed "pathologies" sometimes come to be recognized as lifestyle choices or even normal biological conditions. Homosexuality used to be considered an illness by the medical profession, but today that is no longer the case.

Conversely, moving one's legs around in the middle of the night was not recognized fifty years ago as a mental disorder. Today, however, "Restless Legs Syndrome" (RLS) has an entry in the latest edition of the *Diagnostic Statistical Manual of Mental Disorders* (*DSM*). A wide range of medications are said by their manufacturers to address this "ailment," making it entirely possible for a person to conclude on the basis of a television commercial that he or she suffers from RLS and requires psychotropic medication. Similarly, suggestible persons who avoid parties for one reason or another (shyness, a preference for solitude, etc.) may be persuaded by advertisements alone to believe that they suffer from "Social Anxiety Disorder" (SAD). Again, shortly after a massive push by drug companies to influence public school administrators through the distribution of "scientific" survey batteries, difficult-to-manage children came to be pathologized as well. By now, many millions of them (including a disproportionately large number of foster children, whose medications are paid for by the government) have been prescribed Ritalin and other stimulant drugs, under the assumption that their unruly behavior is symptomatic of a disease: Attention Deficit Hyperactivity Disorder (ADHD).

What has become a profound paradigm shift in modern medicine can be traced to the launch in 1987 and proactive marketing of Prozac for many years. Setting the stage for what was to become a major cultural transformation, many self-styled "scientifically minded" doctors had become disenchanted with Freudian analysis and other forms of "talk therapy." They were easily persuaded to believe that the mind was nothing more and nothing less than the brain, a physical organ the ailments of which could and should be addressed through chemical means. The swift ascendance of the new "biological psychiatry," propelled forward by what were touted as breakthroughs in the pharmaceutical industry, has had effects which ramify through all areas of human life.

Since the launch of Prozac and a panoply of other psychotropic drugs shortly thereafter, the labeling and cataloging of mental illnesses in the ever-proliferating pages of the *DSM* transformed from a more casual endeavor to categorize and organize various symptoms to an unquestioned gospel now embraced by countless medical doctors. Many physicians have no credentials in psychiatry but began prescribing psychiatric medications, as they became readily available, to their regular patients dealing with the ordinary troubles associated with life in human society. An array of psychological states formerly considered normal have been pathologized in tandem with a steady stream of new drug launches. This transformation has been propelled forward through the adoption by hospital and insurance company administrators of the *DSM* as the authoritative reference for determining which treatments to approve.

Difficult to believe though it may be, pharmaceutical companies today synthesize new drugs and then set out to identify novel "diseases" which they can be used to treat. Like all for-profit companies, they use every means at their disposal to ensure that their products succeed. When a product's patent is set to expire, an assiduous effort is undertaken to identify new applications which can be used to secure a patent extension. One noteworthy example was the rebranding of Prozac — generic fluoxetine hydrochloride — as *Sarafem*, which was then marketed in a pink-and-lavender capsule as a "new" drug said to address a newly identified disease, Premenstrual Dysphoric Disorder, or PMDD. Regardless of what one may think about the fact that 25% (or more) of Americans now regularly take psychotropic medications, the opioid crisis initiated by extremely aggressive ploys to sell highly addictive prescription pain pills serves as a stark reminder that marketers are concerned above all with pushing product.

In some ways, none of this is new. Snake oil salesmen and purveyors of so-called panaceas have existed since time immemorial. Prudent people will pause before purchasing (much less ingesting) any product, guided by the ever-handy precept *Caveat Emptor!* In view of the ongoing opioid crisis, set in motion by the rampant overprescription of highly addictive narcotic drugs, many consumers are likely aware that drug companies pay representatives to peddle their products to doctors. What remains less known is that they also hire ghostwriters to pen journal articles, and scientists to design and fund clinical trials, the results of which remain their prerogative to publish or, in the case of negative results, to withhold.[154]

What by now has moved beyond a paradigm shift to constitute a pharmaceutical industry revolution has been marked by four distinct stages, which was perhaps predictable, given what has been going on since 1987. Having first wooed doctors directly through the use of representatives sent out to medical practices to talk up new products and distribute free samples, pharmaceutical companies next captured professional journals and regulatory bodies such as the FDA and the CDC. Medical research is extremely expensive to carry out, and massive funding provided by the ever-more profitable drug industry to universities and research centers further ensured that studies likely to receive financial support — those with profit potential — were naturally pursued. This infiltration into professional, regulatory, and research organizations created a direct feedback loop, whereby clinical physicians (not themselves researchers) were persuaded by institutional authorities to use the products promoted by them. The third stage of this revolution involved wooing patients, through direct-to-consumer advertising, to ask their doctors to prescribe products to them, thus creating a further feedback loop, given that doctors have financial incentives for retaining their patients.

The next logical step in this quest to maximize profit by all means necessary was to infiltrate and capture governments themselves. Governments alone, after all, have the power to *force* their citizenry to do what they want them to do, by threatening a variety of punishments should they fail to acquiesce to their decrees. By making non-compliance with their dictates *illegal*, governments can coerce their populace to do anything and everything, from sacrificing their very own lives in ill-begotten wars, to undergoing experimental treatments of which they have no medical need. Once merely hypothetical, the latter scenario — what is tantamount to *medical fascism* — has been realized in a disturbing number of countries since 2020.

Looking at what has transpired from the perspective of marketing alone, we can see that rather than appealing only to doctors and patients, pharmaceutical companies have now secured seats at the table with government leaders, who have been persuaded to purchase millions of their remedies to distribute "free" to their citizenry. In fact, the entire apparatus undergirding perceptions of the global COVID-19 pandemic — from stickers to masks to tests — has involved a complex nexus of companies contracted by governments, analogous to the symbiosis between government and military industry. President Biden, who interestingly enough holds the record for presidential campaign contributions received from the pharmaceutical industry,[155] recently purchased 1 billion at-home COVID-19 test kits[156] and 400 million N95 masks[157] to be distributed from late January 2022. This initiative virtually guarantees that prevailing perceptions of a "health emergency" will persist at least until Pfizer's new "variant-ready" shot is ready for distribution in March 2022, according to CEO Albert Bourla.[158]

Collaboration between the pharmaceutical industry and governments is not new. Pro-prescription forces captured the Veterans Administration (VA) many years ago. Perhaps the ever-chipper Donald "Stuff Happens" Rumsfeld deserves some credit in this regard, as he chaired pharmaceutical giant G. D. Searle & Company before serving as defense secretary under George W. Bush. In any case, throughout the "War on Terror," soldiers and veterans suffering from PTSD were prescribed massive quantities of psychiatric medications. Even in the face of an epidemic of suicides, which has only grown worse over time, troops continue to be offered cocktails of drugs, not talk therapy, to help them to cope with their psychological distress.[159]

Another example of obvious influence by the pharmaceutical industry has been the widespread marketing by governments of flu vaccines with middling efficacy[160] to their populations, with "free" shots made readily available to everyone just by walking into the local drugstore. In the case of COVID-19, a novel mRNA technology never before tested on human beings was labeled a *vaccine* — before knowing whether it prevented infection and transmission — and marketed on behalf of the manufacturers by governments themselves.

Given this background, it may seem at first glance that what we are witnessing constitutes a continuum in pharmaceutical company influence. In reality, however, it is not a quantitative but a qualitative leap from persuasive advertising (even when misleading) to government coercion. Nonetheless, having come to believe that the government has their best interests in mind, many citizens have been persuaded to go along with whatever measures their leaders impose, up to and including obligatory enrollment in experimental trials.

Somehow oblivious to the Nuremberg Code (see Appendix B), many Western democratic countries, including France, Germany, Austria, Italy, Belgium, Canada, Australia, and New Zealand, have now instituted mandates requiring their citizens to undergo injection of an experimental substance as a condition on their participation in civil society. People in these countries are being refused entry to social venues and retail stores, and even forbidden from working, if they do not present a health "passport" documenting that they have undergone the COVID-19 treatment manufactured by firms such as Pfizer and Moderna. Further coercive measures, affecting nearly everyone everywhere, have included the denial of the freedom to travel to most countries on the planet without first presenting required health "credentials" and in many cases submitting to an inconvenient and expensive period of quarantine. In some places, internment camps have been erected to house persons exposed to COVID-19 and who refuse to undergo the prescribed "treatment" for a disease which kills less than 1% of those infected and which specifically targets elderly persons already suffering from serious health problems.

In the face of the harsh restrictions, which are being applied even to the members of cohorts at minimal risk, some citizens have persisted in resisting and are now facing hefty fines and penalties — including unemployment — for their refusal to comply. In truth, these dissidents, far from being criminals, simply disagree with the government's risk-benefit analysis regarding the wisdom of ingesting this particular "remedy," which we now know, from data in Israel and elsewhere, prevents neither infection nor transmission of the original virus and may have no value whatsoever in the case of the Omicron variant. Logically enough (to anyone familiar with basic concepts of evolution), the virus appears by now to have mutated so as to evade the spike protein antibodies created in response to the foreign substance coded for by the mRNA injections. Vaccine enthusiasts continue nonetheless to rally for the inoculation of everyone everywhere with follow-up booster shots of the elixir created to address the original virus, not the mutant variants.

Marketing deployed by governments is propaganda, the promotion of ideas and ideology. What we are now witnessing, however, unprecedented in history, is an amalgamation of pharmaceutical interests with governments to forge a pharma-techno-fascist regime requiring "health passports" of citizens in order to be able to participate in society. Following the tried-and-true playbook for military intervention, leaders and pundits have claimed that we are on a "war" footing in "combating" COVID-19, which is taken to entail both that "the evil enemy" must be defeated and that the citizenry must make sacrifices to see that this be done. Over the course of two years, what began as "Stay home two weeks to flatten the curve!" has transmogrified to "Undergo mandatory injection of a foreign substance at regular intervals as specified by the relevant authorities — or else face ostracism and criminal penalties!"

This fourth stage of the pharma revolution should be recognized for what it is: a veritable coup, for entire governments have now been captured by the drug industry. But if most countries still prohibit direct-to-consumer advertising of drugs, how did this coup come about? The primary tactic in securing mass compliance among large portions of the populace in countries all over the world has been the control of news programs by the pharmaceutical companies, which serve as financial sponsors of major networks. When the news is underwritten by vested interests in a particular industry, then it becomes difficult to distinguish facts from propaganda, just as in the case of wars promoted by television newscasters under a guise of patriotism, when in fact they receive funding from for-profit companies in the military industry.

People are now being told by leaders and their spokespersons, including the so-called journalists who parrot them, that they must undergo whatever medical treatment their government dictates, as specified by public health organizations which have been altogether colonized by the pharmaceutical industry. These significant conflicts of interest are ignored by pundits and the populace, just as in wartime, on the grounds that only those "in the know," that is, with ties to the industry in question, are qualified to offer competent advice. This same line of reasoning has been incessantly repeated throughout the mainstream media in calls for the censorship of divergent opinions, even among fully credentialed medical doctors and researchers.

The claim to be fighting a "war" against COVID-19 opened the door to not only censorship but also quasi-martial law and precisely the sorts of lockdowns, quarantines, and curfews we have seen implemented in the name of public health, even as statistical data emerged to refute what many had hoped would be the efficacy of such measures. When social distancing and masking failed to stop the virus, pharmaceutical companies came forward with their usual claims of magical cures for the scourge of this new disease.

The history of the ascendance of the drug industry since 1987 reveals that pharma marketers are among the savviest beasts around, and the persuasion of government officials to *coerce* their citizenry to undergo medical treatments should be acknowledged for what it is: a brilliant marketing scheme. Having already reaped the benefits of their massive campaigns to lure as many people into the use of "comfort" and "lifestyle" drugs as they possibly could — with targets ranging the gamut from infants to nonagenarians, and by now including even family pets — pharma firms have during the fourth stage of this revolution capitalized on the appearance of COVID-19 on the scene to peddle their wares to nearly every living person on the planet. The collaboration of Pfizer, Moderna, and other companies with governments has been deceptively depicted as philanthropic, which contradicts not only the purely profit-driven nature of publicly traded companies but also the heavy-handed, coercive measures being deployed by governments against people who decline treatment.

One must admit that labeling the novel mRNA therapy, which is helpful to those who are vulnerable to COVID-19, a *vaccine* was itself a slick trick, for it not only offered the product companies indemnity from legal prosecution in the event of adverse effects (under the PREP Act[161]) but also made it possible to lump anyone who resisted into the class of *Untermenschen* derided throughout the media and by an uncanny coalition of celebrities — ranging from Howard Stern to Stephen King to Jennifer Aniston to Neil Young — as *anti-vaxxers*. The self-righteous pro-vax mob may have no actual understanding of the distinction between absolute risk reduction (ARR) and relative risk reduction (RRR),[162] an ignorance capitalized upon by marketers of the various shots being provided "free" to citizens, but they do know whom to believe: Fauci & Co.

The initial marketing blitz for the shots boasted a miraculous 95% efficacy rate in avoiding severe illness and death, which was slyly suggested to apply to all persons, when in fact it applied much more narrowly to those vulnerable to the virus, particularly advanced seniors who also suffer from multiple health problems, making it difficult for their bodies to defeat the virus. The vast majority of younger and healthier persons are capable of avoiding hospitalization and death without any treatment whatsoever. Yet the initial "95% efficacy" claim has been used in calls for people from all age groups, even those at no significant risk from the virus, to undergo vaccination. When Biden's press secretary, Jen Psaki, despite being fully vaccinated, became infected with and recovered from COVID-19, she sang Pfizer's favorite refrain, that her illness was mild only as a result of the vaccine. Straight from the government's mouth, this is manifestly disinformation, the equivalent of a marketing jingle, given the low statistical probability that a healthy woman in her forties might suffer severe illness from or be killed by COVID-19.

It is also disinformation, continually pumped out by government propagandists, to mislabel people who raise specific, science-based concerns about the experimental mRNA treatments as *anti-vaxxers*, even when they have objections neither to time-tested medical treatments nor to vaccines in general. On the basis of such propaganda, those who refuse to comply are being more and more sternly admonished for shirking what is painted as every citizen's duty, and because public health authorities such as Anthony Fauci continue to label dissenters themselves as purveyors of "disinformation," much of the populace is inclined to fall in line, chiming in with government propagandists to denounce anyone who dares to disagree.

A variety of other marketing tricks have been deployed throughout the Coronapocalypse as well, from the denial of the reality of natural immunity, to the focus on anecdotal cases of outliers who supposedly demonstrate the vulnerability of everyone — in every age and health cohort — to the virus.

Needless to say, outliers on the vaccine adverse effects curve are entirely ignored. Similarly, the very fact that the average age of COVID-19 victims in some places has been higher than their life expectancy is not a topic of discussion on any of the programs relentlessly promoting universal vaccination.

Just as antiwar activists are denounced by hawks as traitors and cowards, the push to mandate medical treatments at the behest of those advising the government has involved characterizing citizens who refuse to comply as ignorant, stupid, selfish, and even evil. Fear is a powerful motivator to action, as is demonstrated by both the history of warfare and the history of drug marketing. Tell people that the enemy (whether a foreign government or a disease) is going to kill them, and they will volunteer to kill whoever the enemy is claimed to be, or at the very least pay others to do so. If some of their fellow human beings are the vehicle of evil, then they, too, will need to be eliminated or contained.

The twist in this fourth stage of the pharma revolution is that now unvaccinated persons have been cast as "the enemy," with all that this implies, up to and including calls to restrict their movement and access to social spheres. Thus we find leaders such as Canadian Prime Minister Justin Trudeau asking unfacetiously, with no apparent irony, whether unvaccinated persons should be "tolerated."[163] The president of France, Emmanuel Macron, has expressed similar scorn for the unvaccinated inhabitants of his land, claiming that he will do whatever is necessary to force them to comply with the medical mandates severely restricting their activities since the summer of 2021.[164] It matters perhaps little at this point whether functional sociopaths in high places became that way naturally or through the ingestion of psychotropic drugs. They are who they are. Our task remains to defend our shrinking freedoms from those who would take them away.

The attempt of ostensibly democratic governments to usurp the bodily autonomy of their citizenry through the use of propaganda and coercion is an appalling development, but it is not yet too late to disabuse those led astray. Recognizing the pharmaceutical industry revolution of the past thirty-five years is the key to understanding how we arrived where we are today.

18. Whatever Happened to Medical Ethics?

March 10, 2022
Holladay, Utah

I recall being shown in grade school a series of short films about the danger of seemingly friendly men who drove popsicle trucks and tried to lure young children into accepting free treats. We were sternly instructed to stay far, far away from such people. How the world has changed.

Today we have political leaders with no knowledge of our personal health situation asking us to accept injections of experimental substances for the simple reason that they have been told by their advisers (also ignorant of our circumstances) that it would be good for us to do. It is a bizarre, even absurd, idea that healthy persons should agree to inject any substance at the behest of people who know nothing about them. In fact, it is the opposite of what we were trained to believe throughout childhood, when everyone was strictly warned not to accept gifts from strangers, least of all drugs with unknown effects.

Fellow citizens, something sinister is afoot. Many people have been persuaded, through mountains of propaganda and divisive rhetoric, that the government can decree what substances its citizens must ingest. This is unprecedented in the history of democratic society and represents a rejection of the patient-centered paradigm of medical ethics. Bodily autonomy is no small thing, and yet the leaders of many governments have pushed relentlessly to strip it away, insisting, in direct contradiction to the Nuremberg Code (see Appendix B), that you do not have a right to decline the injection of a substance into your very own body.

COVID-19 "vaccination" has been made a requirement on participation in civil society in many countries. You may not travel to most parts of the world without first demonstrating that you have complied with the reigning vaccination regimen. (Last I checked, U.S. citizens are allowed to travel to a grand total of five countries without providing health documents.) This is not, as some may claim, a matter of mere inconvenience, for people are being through these policies *conditioned to believe* that governments have the right and the authority to mandate medical procedures. If healthy people must now share their medical records with government officials, what else can they be required to do? The digital identification system being implemented can be deployed far more generally to restrict the activities of persons who dare even to disagree with the government. Consider what happened recently in Canada.

When Prime Minister Justin Trudeau invoked emergency powers to freeze the bank accounts of anyone, regardless of vaccination status, who donated to the trucker convoy, he demonstrated for all to see how dangerous the present situation has become. To criminalize dissent in this way is to open the door to a system of totalitarian tyranny, where people said by government officials to hold "unacceptable" opinions can be stopped in their tracks by a variety of means. In some ways, all of this has served as a test to see what people will accept. The results are disconcerting, to say the least.

The Freedom Truck Convoy protest in Canada was portrayed by the media as a gigantic nuisance, with nearly no attention given to the rational basis of the dissent: a rejection of the notion that truckers, who spend most of their day alone inside the cab of their vehicle, should be required to undergo injection of a foreign substance which they themselves have already concluded is not in their best interests. Some among the vaccine hesitant are persons who do not, as a matter of prudence, volunteer to serve in trials of new medications, and certainly not when they are not suffering from any disease. Others are persons who already survived COVID-19 and base their refusal to undergo inoculation on the concepts of "immunity" and "vaccine" which held sway for their entire lives — until the Coronapocalypse. These people quite reasonably accept what before 2020 was a widely held precept among doctors and patients alike: *Do not undergo unnecessary medical procedures or accept prescriptions for drugs which you do not need.*

It used to be that anything labeled a "vaccine" could be depended on to prevent infection and transmission of a disease, which the novel mRNA shots do not. It used to be equally obvious that anyone who had already survived a disease had no need to take a vaccine against it, for he had already developed antibodies and T-cells to combat it naturally. It stands to reason that, if natural immunity does not protect a person, then neither does a vaccine which depends on natural immunity in order to work. That so many, even educated, people do not recognize this obvious implication is best, and perhaps only, explained by the discombobulation induced by the government's assiduous propaganda campaign, which instilled an irrational fear of death into the populace over a period of two years. President Biden's cheery Christmastime 2021 salutation, that unvaccinated persons could expect "a winter of severe illness and death," was typical in this regard.

Many of the people who have declined the shot studied the statistics and concluded that, given their likelihood of surviving the virus, they preferred to bet on their own immune system. In truth, no one should be in the position of having to explain his own medical choices to anyone else, which makes it all the more unbelievable that people are being asked to accept injections of substances with unknown long-term side effects, and for which the manufacturers have been granted legal immunity in the event of any, even proximate, adverse events. This blanket indemnity has been conferred upon the product companies by the very governments which not only purchased the shots but also funded their research and development.

People the world over have been complying with nonsensical measures — such as wearing cloth masks with no prophylactic benefit against airborne viruses, and being injected with spike protein mRNA when they already survived COVID-19 — simply in order to be able to keep their jobs and lead some semblance of a life. In complying, they have tacitly renounced their right not to do ridiculous things at the behest of politically appointed officials. It's as though these people have already signed a form granting the government the authority to require them to do whatever it wants them to do, freedom be damned. This radical transformation in the norms of society has been rationalized under a "public health" pretext, despite its rejection of the most basic principles of medical ethics upheld since time immemorial.

Until 2020, doctors were taught that patients must be treated as human beings with the capacity to assess the risks and benefits of any prospective medication and decide for themselves whether taking it is something which they wish to do. Only for persons who are not fully responsible, such as children, elderly persons with diminished cognitive capacities, and the mentally ill, are health decisions made by their legal guardians instead. For the leader of a nation to assume the right and power to decide whom to medicate is to render society the equivalent of a psychiatric ward, filled with people incapable of thinking for themselves. To medicate such persons against their will can only be predicated on the assumption that they are incompetent to make such decisions.

The grand irony in the present case is that ostensibly free citizens have been told by their governments that they must follow the decrees of their elected officials and their associated appointees. But if the citizens are truly incapable of making medical decisions for themselves, then they are equally incapable of selecting their leaders. In other words, the legitimacy of any leader who claims to be able to force medical treatments on his citizens is undermined by the implication that those very same people are not responsible for their own choices, including their election of the leader in question.

Nonetheless, over the past two years, heads of state have not only offered COVID-19 shots to their citizens, but further mandated that they undergo this novel mRNA treatment, never before tested on human beings, and of which many of them have no need, according to all available statistical data. The leaders claim that the "vaccines" are free, when in fact billions of doses were purchased using citizens' tax dollars. As a result of the large stockpiles in many First World countries, where everyone who wished to take the shot has already been provided with the opportunity to do so, leaders such as Canada's Justin Trudeau, France's Emmanuel Macron, and New Zealand's Jacinda Ardern have grown increasingly intolerant of anyone who disagrees with them, expressing overt irritation and disdain toward those who persist in refusing to submit to the medical treatments purchased by the leaders on their behalf.

Political leaders are, in the vast majority of cases, total strangers to us, persons about whom we know only that they managed to get elected, by hook or by crook. Why in the world should anyone accept medical advice, much less orders to undergo injection of an experimental remedy, from a politician? It boggles the mind. In the specific case of the COVID-19 vaccines, there are multiple reasons for exercising caution. It is one thing to trust someone about whom one knows nothing, and, for some people, the default position is charitably to confer upon others the benefit of the doubt. It is quite another to trust parties with a demonstrated record of deception and fraud.

As the opioid crisis continues to play out across the United States, with record numbers of overdoses, it is difficult to understand why anyone should now trust the FDA when it comes to COVID-19. After all, regulators themselves condoned for years the pharmaceutical giants' grossly misleading campaign to massively increase prescriptions of narcotics to anyone and everyone for anything. The catastrophic results have been the creation of millions of addicts and the direct or indirect cause of hundreds of thousands of associated overdose deaths. Yet pharma-sponsored media pundits and puppets such as Anthony Fauci and CDC Director Rochelle Walensky, unfazed by the simultaneous overdose epidemic currently underway, have continued to gush that the FDA represents "the gold standard" for safety determinations about the substances which people can and should put into their bodies.

Taking irony to an entirely new level, the opioid overdose epidemic was exacerbated by the lockdowns rationalized under a bogus pretext of stemming the tide of the COVID-19 pandemic. As a result of the lockdowns, many people were rendered hopeless by the sudden proscription of normal social activities. Some among them lost their means of livelihood, and even their homes, as can be seen in the ever-expanding tent encampments all over the United States. But those lockdowns, which proved to be deadly, were in fact imposed at the recommendation of "public health experts," providing further grounds for skepticism in following their advice.

In the first decade of what became the opioid crisis, regulators consistently and persuasively supported pharmaceutical company marketers as they preposterously insisted that powerful narcotic pills were not addictive. Likewise, during the Coronapocalypse, public health officials contributed decisively to the false portrayal of what was made to seem the imminent virus-induced death of everyone, when in fact only a small percentage of the population was truly vulnerable. Traumatized and terrified citizens lined up by the millions when the vaccines became available, even though most of them were never going to suffer severe illness, much less die, from COVID-19.

The mental health crisis caused by the fearmongering campaign and the lockdowns, which had no positive effect on the virus death toll, did lead to a large increase in non-virus deaths — including not only drug overdoses but also suicides. The fact that routine screenings were postponed as a result of the lockdowns, leading to thousands of late diagnoses of cancer and other life-threatening diseases, reveals that the public health establishment, in pushing its monomaniacal vaccine agenda, was willing to *kill* people, yet more compelling evidence (beyond the opioid overprescription debacle) of full capture by the pharmaceutical industry. This hypothesis also provides the best explanation for the refusal of officials to promote non-vaccine therapies and drugs not under patent, as Robert F. Kennedy, Jr., has ably documented in his disturbing tale of moral horror, *The Real Anthony Fauci:*

Bill Gates, Big Pharma, and the Global War on Democracy and Public Health (2021),[165] which every person affected by the Coronapocalypse should read.

When questioned about the negative effects of the lockdowns, Dr. Fauci explained in his usual dismissive manner that he does not offer "economic advice," only public health guidance. But, as the authors of the Great Barrington Declaration (see Appendix A) rightly observed, there were many other aspects of public health to consider in weighing policy options in response to the appearance and spread of the COVID-19 virus. The Great Barrington Declaration doctors and epidemiologists were denounced, discredited, and censored when they issued their warnings back in October 2020. Now that their many concerns have been validated statistically, those who pushed for what proved to be destructive policies blithely deny any responsibility for the damage done. In a meritocratic world, the people whose policies failed would be fired. Instead, they are invited back as "experts" to opine on mainstream media news network programs sponsored by the pharmaceutical industry. This pharma-friendly, biased coverage of the pandemic explains why and how many people continue to regard Pfizer, in particular, as a world leader in confronting the scourge of COVID-19.

Pfizer paid the largest fine for healthcare fraud in the history of the world. Pfizer misleadingly claimed that its new COVID-19 vaccine offered 95% efficacy against a virus which most people already had a 99.5% chance of surviving. Recently released documents reveal that Pfizer knew that the lethality of COVID-19 was similar to that of the seasonal flu. Pfizer announced that a new shot to address the Omicron variant was in the works and would be available in March 2022, while simultaneously continuing to insist that everyone needed to get a third — or even fourth — dose of the original shot, rebranded as "the booster," as well.

Now that Pfizer has been court ordered to release its vaccine trial safety data, the billions of people who took the shot will at last have the missing half of "informed consent" which the naysayers have been waiting for all along.[166] With regard to adverse effects, vaccine enthusiasts have relentlessly insisted that the VAERS (Vaccine Adverse Events Reporting System) database is undependable and that no one should believe the thousands of reports of deaths, permanent injuries, heart attacks, miscarriages, etc., claimed to have ensued after injection, all of which supposedly mistook correlation for causation.

Informed consent is arguably the most fundamental requirement of medical ethics, and now that Pfizer's own data is being made public, there seems to be no way to deny the reality of the many reported adverse effects which have been consistently minimized by the media in efforts to maximize vaccine uptake. Yet vaccine hesitancy continues to be depicted as not prudential but selfish and evil, despite the statistical reality that some countries with very low vaccination rates had better cumulative health outcomes than wealthy countries which invested in billions of shots. Apparently unwilling or unable to face the statistics, many citizens persist in their pro-vaccine posture, prepared to undergo injection of whatever the government decrees on a schedule determined by public health authorities who are either incredibly incompetent or (*vel*) completely coopted.

Now, it might seem that, if the vaccines actually worked, then the case for imposing them on unwilling persons would be stronger. The canned response to those who reject mandatory vaccination is that some people cannot survive the shots, because they are immunocompromised, so everyone who can be vaccinated must be vaccinated, in order to protect the vulnerable. Anyone who refuses to undergo the treatment is selfish and despicable, an enemy of society, and should therefore be ostracized and even criminalized. In reality, this line of reasoning is not upheld in any other area where some people may be harmed if they choose to comport themselves in ways which put them at special risk because of factors peculiar to them.

No one claims that all restaurants must stop selling pasta because persons suffering from Celiac disease may be accidentally exposed to gluten if their server mixes up the orders or forgets to request gluten-free pasta from the kitchen. No one calls for a moratorium on contact sports on the grounds that hemophiliacs exist. In all such cases, people with special vulnerabilities (or their caretakers) are expected to exercise extraordinary vigilance. Why should the vulnerability of elderly, immunocompromised, and obese persons be accepted as the basis for shutting down all of society and mandating medical procedures for people who neither want nor need them?

Some will retort that COVID-19 is an infectious disease. But the lethality of COVID-19 is similar to that of the seasonal flu, which is also caused by transmissible viruses. Before 2020, no political leaders coerced their populations to submit to flu shots with mediocre efficacy on the grounds that thousands of elderly and frail persons might die should they contract the flu. The sobering truth is that more people died of COVID-19 after the mass vaccination program than before.

In any case, that the treatment were efficacious — a *vaccine* in the traditional sense, which reliably prevented both infection and transmission for decades (not months), and offered significant risk reduction (not ~1%, as the mRNA shots do for most people) — would constitute only a *necessary* condition on the rational decision of any person to agree to injection. According to longstanding norms governing the practice of ethical medicine, the sufficient condition for a patient to take a drug or undergo a treatment recommended by his physician is that the person should choose to do so — whatever his reasons may be.

Just as in the case of wars claimed to be necessary by officials, it was the media-generated fear of death throughout the Coronapocalypse which led people to accept whatever their governments said, even when it flew in the face of decades of knowledge about immunology. Given the influence exerted by pharmaceutical company lobbyists on politicians in the United States, no one should be surprised that pro-pharma firm policies have in every case held sway. Vaccine mandates were implemented by many leaders and imposed by private companies at the state and local level, despite the U.S. Supreme Court's rejection of the federal OSHA mandate.

The Supreme Court did, however, uphold the federal mandate on healthcare workers, which led to the firing of thousands of persons for refusing to undergo vaccination. This unfortunate ruling was based in part on the manifestly false assumption pumped out by public health and other government officials on behalf of the pharmaceutical industry, that previously infected and already recovered workers constituted a danger to their coworkers and patients. That the Supreme Court's decision was based on disinformation — including the slippery equivocation in the use of the word *vaccine*, which until 2020 meant a substance which prevented infection and transmission — has gone largely ignored by the media.

Dozens of scientific, peer-reviewed studies have demonstrated that persons who already recovered from COVID-19 have more robust and longer-lasting immunity than the mRNA shots can provide. Falsehoods such as that asymptomatic carriers were the drivers of the pandemic have by now been thoroughly debunked. Doctors who have served as industry shills, encouraging pregnant women, children, and already recovered patients to serve as subjects in pharmaceutical trials of treatments of which they had no need, and securing the consent of patients to undergo vaccination without providing them with full information, should be shunned no less than the doctors who propelled the opioid crisis forward through the overprescription of narcotic pills falsely portrayed as nonaddictive.

It goes without saying that forced vaccination violates the libertarian's Non-Aggression Principle (NAP). Sticking a needle into a person's body against his will is a flagrant act of violence, the moral equivalent of pharmaceutical rape.[167] Both bribery and coercion are immoral means by which to undermine personal autonomy in influencing medical choices. If we are to remain free and retain control of our own bodies, the politicians who deployed and supported any of the misleading tactics used since 2020 to undermine the rights of citizens, in the name of public health but at the expense of medical ethics, must be relieved of their positions by voters at the earliest possible opportunity.

19. The Necro-Neologism of Lethal Legal Experts

March 28, 2022
Holladay, Utah

The power of language is magical to behold. Through the mere pronouncement of words, people can be persuaded to do what they would never have thought to do, left to their own devices. The playbook with the most success in this regard is that of war. When people are "informed" that they and their families are in mortal danger, they may and often will acquiesce to any and all policies which government authorities claim to be necessary in order to protect them.

Young people can be coaxed into killing complete strangers who never did anything personally to them. Citizens can be brainwashed to believe that suitably labeled persons can and indeed must be denied any and all human rights. When the stakes are claimed to be life and death, even apparently intelligent people can be goaded to accept that the mere possession of a divergent opinion is evil, and the expression of dissent a crime. The use of military weapons to execute obviously innocent, entirely innocuous civilians, including children, suddenly becomes permissible, so long as the victims have been labeled "collateral damage." All any of this takes is to identify "the enemy" as evil.

In centuries past, "the laws of war" were said to require the humane treatment of enemy soldiers. They were diagnosed as suffering from "invincible ignorance," misled and mistaken about the dispute said to necessitate recourse to war, but still acknowledged as persons capable of being courageous combatants who found themselves through historical fortuity on the wrong side. An enemy soldier was to be provided with the opportunity to lay down his weapon and surrender in order to save his own life. Disarmed or incapacitated soldiers were not to be executed by their captors, for they had already been neutralized and posed no more danger than unarmed civilians. Prisoners of war were to be treated as human beings, and when they were tortured or summarily executed, this constituted a war crime. Such "laws of war," which form the basis of international agreements, including the Geneva Conventions, have needless to say often been flouted, but, in theory, they were to be upheld by civilized people.

Neologism and Redefinition in the War on Terror

After the terrorist attacks of September 11, 2001, political leaders and government officials proclaimed that "everything changed." The Bush administration legal team deployed linguistic innovation to issue in an entirely new era of warfare, wherein "the laws of war" would remain in place, but they would be inapplicable to entire classes of human beings. Jihadist soldiers for radical Islamist causes were labeled *unlawful enemy combatants*, whose "unlawful" status was said to imply that they were protected by neither international norms such as the Geneva Conventions nor the laws of civil society.

Under this pretext, terrorist suspects were tortured while held captive at prisons in Guantánamo Bay, Abu Ghraib, and Bagram, in addition to many black sites around the world.[168] Ever keen to cover their tracks, the Central Intelligence Agency (CIA) also flatly denied that they ever tortured anyone, by redefining as *enhanced interrogation techniques* the abusive practices inflicted on hundreds, if not thousands, of men in an effort to extract from them actionable intelligence. And just in case any of this "logic" was called into question by pesky human rights advocates, Bush administration officials also derided the Geneva Conventions as "quaint."

The "peace candidate" Barack Obama was elected in 2008 on the promise to rein in the excesses of the Bush administration, including what Obama characterized as the "dumb" war on Iraq. The new president publicly denounced "enhanced interrogation techniques" as torture but then proceeded to take linguistic neologism to an entirely new level by not only redefining *assassination* as *targeted killing* but also labeling any suspect eliminated through the use of lethal drones as an *Enemy Killed in Action* (EKIA).

The slaughtered "soldiers" were assumed to be guilty of possible complicity in future possible crimes, a preposterous position never fully grasped by Obama's devotees, who somehow failed to recognize that the specific implement used to kill does not distinguish various types of homicide from one another, morally speaking. The extrajudicial execution of individual human beings in civil society is illegal, but the Obama administration maintained that the targeting of suspicious persons and their associates in lands far away was perfectly permissible. According to the drone warriors, using missiles launched from drones sufficed to transform acts of intentional, premeditated homicide (formerly known as "assassination") into "acts of war."

The entire drone program, whether within or far from areas of active hostilities (i.e., war zones), was portrayed by Obama and his administration as just another facet of "just war." Blinded to the moral atrocity of this new lethal-centric approach to dealing with suspected enemies, whereby they would be executed rather than taken prisoner, Obama's loyal supporters blithely embraced the propaganda according to which he was a *smart warrior*. After demonstrating his death creds to the satisfaction of hawks, by killing not only Osama bin Laden but also U.S. citizen Anwar al-Awlaki, who had been suspected of complicity in factional terrorism, Obama was reelected for a second term in 2012, despite having summarily executed thousands of men — mostly brown-skinned, unnamed, and unarmed — located in their own civil societies, far from any U.S. citizen, and in clear violation of the Geneva Conventions.

The deft deployment of two simple words, *immediate* and *imminent*, played a key role in allowing Obama to get away with murder,[169] even of U.S. citizens such as Anwar al-Awlaki and his sixteen-year-old son, Abdulrahman al-Awlaki. Guided by drone-killing czar John Brennan, Obama's lawyers calmly explained in public addresses and official documents that suspects who posed imminent threats to the United States could be targeted by lethal drones because an *imminent* threat did not imply *immediacy*. In other words, they could be killed even when they were currently unarmed and living in their own civil society, surrounded by family members and friends, and even when the future crime of which they were vaguely suspected was merely hypothetical and therefore had no specific date.

When targets were "nominated" for execution, the administration operated under the assumption that they were guilty unless specific information was brought forth to demonstrate their innocence. The victims themselves obviously could not do this, initially, because they were not informed that they were being targeted and, later, because they were dead. Meanwhile, local residents and journalists on the ground who knew these people's names and dared to assert that the victims were not terrorists were either denounced as propagandists or cast as misguided persons hoodwinked by the rhetoric of jihadists.

As the death toll mounted, outspoken critics in the vicinity of the missile strikes became progressively more terrified of being themselves eliminated for seeming to support terrorist groups. Their concerns were not unfounded, for they risked being affixed with the lethal label *associate* and added to hit lists for execution if they dared to question the drone warriors' narrative. This oppressive climate served to suppress dissent from the U.S. government's official story of what had been done, even among locals who witnessed the grisly scenes where entirely innocent community members were incinerated by missiles launched from drones.

Neologism and Redefinition in the Prescription Narcotic Addiction Crisis

Improbably enough, the very same two words, *imminent* and *immediate*, used by the Obama legal team to invert the presumption of innocence to a presumption of guilt in the case of terrorist suspects located abroad, proved to be deadly in an entirely different context during the twenty-first century as well.

The causes of the sudden and shocking increase in the number of narcotics addicts and overdose deaths all over the United States are manifold, but a tidal wave of diversion was made possible by drug-dealer doctors and the notorious "pain clinics" where they plied their trade. Manufacturers produced and pharmacies dispensed billions of pills as demand multiplied in tandem with the creation of more and more new addicts, who could no longer function without narcotics.

Purdue Pharma and the Sackler family are widely regarded as the prime movers of the opioid crisis, having undertaken a highly successful campaign to coax doctors into believing that their patented time-release prescription narcotic Oxycontin was nonaddictive and could be safely provided to patients even for moderate pain. This marketing feat was achieved by influencing key players at the FDA, who not only approved the medication but permitted it to be sold along with a package insert falsely suggesting that it was less prone to abuse than other narcotics.

In its quest to sell as many pills as possible, the pharmaceutical industry repeatedly pivoted to neologize in lethal ways over the two decades following the launch of Oxycontin in 1996. When it emerged that the pills sometimes wore off before the twelve-hour time release period, marketers and sales representatives claimed that those patients were suffering from *breakthrough pain*, the remedy for which was (surprise!) to double their dose. The narcotics marketers indulged in flat-out sophistry when they insisted that patients who appeared to be addicted to their painkillers were in fact suffering from *pseudoaddiction*, the remedy for which was (surprise!) even higher doses of their drugs. As farcical as these arguments may seem in retrospect, with the benefit of hindsight and in the light of the overdose epidemic now running rampant, many doctors appear to have been persuaded to believe that their patients' miserable condition was not indicative of addiction but a manifestation of their ongoing and unbearable pain, the solution to which was to ply them with yet more powerful narcotics.

Pharma-coopted lawmakers were notified of the proliferating addiction problem early on but refused to stop the runaway train by demanding that the FDA cease playing along with Purdue's insane pro-narcotics marketing campaign. Other companies, needless to say, contributed as well, through promulgating the "pain epidemic" propaganda in order to expand the market niche of such products, which had previously been reserved for terminally ill patients. Johnson & Johnson played a causal role in what became the opioid crisis by growing tons of poppies (in Tasmania) to meet the enormous increased industry need for raw opium, without which the billions of pills prescribed could not and would never have been produced.

As the opioid crisis began to become recognized for what it was, the Drug Enforcement Administration (DEA) sought to issue "Immediate Suspension Orders" (ISOs) against the three major drug wholesale distributors to pharmacies: Cardinal Health, McKesson, and AmerisourceBergen. Through issuing such orders, Joe Rannazzisi, the deputy director of the Office of Diversion Control, hoped to halt the ongoing mass shipments of narcotics to retailers such as CVS in cases where the sheer volume of prescriptions could not be explained by ordinary medical practice and so was a clear indication that widespread diversion was underway.

Rannazzisi ended up being hobbled by a team of corporate lawyers and lobbyists who managed to cobble together a new law in 2014 which, despite its beneficent-sounding name, "The Ensuring Patient Access and Effective Drug Enforcement Act" (H.R. 4709), served to protect, above all, drug manufacturers and distributors.[170] The Act rewrote the law already on the books through redefining the *imminent danger* required to issue an ISO to mean "a substantial likelihood of an immediate threat." One of the new Act's enthusiastic promoters, Linden Barber (a former DEA officer and lawyer who had left his government position to represent the drug distributors), persuasively explained on the floor of Congress that "having a clear legal standard is always better." The measure passed unanimously, without a roll call vote, for the simple reason that it sounded like a policy to which no decent person could object. Instead of stemming the tide of the opioid crisis, the Act severely hampered the DEA's ability to issue ISOs, for it was prohibitively difficult for officials to meet the newly stipulated legal standard of *imminence* as requiring *immediacy*.[171]

President Obama signed the Ensuring Patient Access and Effective Drug Enforcement Act of 2014 into law, and the marketing campaign used to promote the use of highly addictive time-release narcotics barreled ahead. The DEA's sudden inability to call a halt to the shipment of tons of narcotics to retailers effectively guaranteed that the number of dependent persons would multiply, as potent prescription pills continued to be diverted for recreational uses, thereby creating more addicts. But more addicts meant more overdoses, not only from the potent pills themselves, but also because the street supplies of heroin to which many users eventually turned were often cut with extremely dangerous fentanyl.[172]

Unfazed by the death tolls, which had already soared to many thousands by 2014, the pharmaceutical giants insisted that the sorry situation of addicts was no argument against helping patients genuinely in pain, who would in fact be wronged if their access to narcotics were curbed. The addicts dropping like flies were painted as solely responsible for their plight, despite ample evidence that many of the overdose victims began as legitimate pain patients, who became aware of their dependency only upon reaching the bottom of their amber vials.

In this way, "everything changed" in the twenty-first century, not only with the "War on Terror," the rebranding of torture, and the normalization of assassination, but also in the pharma-friendly approach to healthcare ushered in by President Barack Obama. By pushing through his signature legislation, the Affordable Care Act (ACA) of 2010, which leftists were led to believe would create a system of socialized medicine (referred to by many as *Obamacare*), the president notoriously bowed to drug makers and the insurance industry, extending to those sectors the very form of crony corporate welfare already enjoyed by companies in the military industry.

Obama's collaboration with pharmaceutical and insurance company executives in crafting the ACA allowed them to secure advantageous pricing arrangements to ensure the maximization of their profits while at the same time massively increasing the sheer volume of sales. The pharmaceutical industry was greatly enriched through the provision of virtually limitless free psychiatric medications to low-income patients through government programs such as Medicaid and Medicare, and to veterans through the VA. Mental health-based disability claims soared, and the sales of SSRIs (selective serotonin reuptake inhibitors), anti-anxiety, atypical anti-psychotic medications, and other psychotropic drugs, including narcotics, increased accordingly. The millions of new prescription medications dispensed to formerly uninsured Americans ended up being paid for by the middle class, who were mandated by law to sign up for Obamacare or else face a hefty tax penalty should they decline to comply.

Despite what may have been Obama's initial good intention — to make healthcare available to uninsured persons — Obamacare ultimately made medical treatment in the United States prohibitively expensive for many middle-class families, whose co-pays, premiums, and deductibles dramatically increased. The new mandatory healthcare program skyrocketed the salaries of health industry executives while pricing drugs and procedures out of reach for many persons who had previously been able to afford them. Millions of people in the United States have filed medical bankruptcy in recent years. In cases where prescription narcotics addicts became uninsured because they lost their jobs, they turned to the streets for their needed drugs, given the impossibility of paying out of pocket for extraordinarily expensive prescription pills.

Given the story of Obamacare, perhaps no one should be surprised that when the Obama administration finally took action to address the opioid epidemic, most of the allocated $1.1 billion was for the alternative medication of already existing addicts.[173] The pharma-friendly approach prevailed once again, encouraging the sale of more and more drugs (such as Suboxone[174]) to help addicts to wean themselves off their narcotics. Obama's dilatory and pro-pill approach to the opioid crisis ultimately generated even more people who, in order to kick their narcotics habit, would need to avail themselves of further pharmaceutical means, effectively trading one drug for another. In other words, both the problem of opioid overprescription, facilitated through Obamacare by providing easy access to narcotics to formerly uninsured persons, and the measures implemented by the Obama administration in response to the overdose epidemic, served to increase pharmaceutical industry profits, at the expense of citizens' lives.

Neologism and Redefinition in the Coronapocalypse

The government's handling of what became the COVID-19 crisis illustrates, too, the very same callous disregard for the well-being of citizens, ironically, by public health officials whose ostensible job it is to protect society from medical threats. Rather than effectively shielding the vulnerable, however, government-imposed policies caused a general decrease in life expectancy for the population as a whole. The many other, less lethal harms, such as the children whose learning was severely compromised during the period of the pandemic, and the creation of a society of persons afraid to interact with others or to go anywhere, cannot be quantified.

That so many persons not vulnerable to COVID-19 ended up succumbing unwittingly to fentanyl-laced drug abuse, having lost their jobs, businesses, and homes, reveals again that the policymakers were focused all along on promoting the interests of their most generous sponsors, not the population whom they were elected to represent. Like the normalization of assassination and the prolongation through legislation of the opioid crisis, the harms done by the political handling of COVID-19 were made possible through neologism.

In earlier times, before the H1N1 swine flu appeared in 2009, the term *pandemic* was reserved for simultaneous outbreaks worldwide involving much higher than usual death rates. Removing the requirement of severity from the definition allowed the use of the term *pandemic* to trigger WHO measures to promote swift vaccine development and distribution. Similarly, in 2020, the new definition was instrumental in causing the lockstep lockdowns of people by governments all over the world.

More recently, the term *vaccine* was also changed. In 2018, the CDC defined the term as:

> a product that *stimulates a person's immune system to produce immunity to a specific disease*, protecting the person from that disease. Vaccines are usually administered through needle injections, but can also be administered by mouth or sprayed into the nose.[175] [my emphasis]

In 2021, the CDC redefined *vaccine* as:

> a preparation that is *used to stimulate the body's immune response against diseases*. Vaccines are usually administered through needle injections, but some can be administered by mouth or sprayed into the nose.[176] [my emphasis]

This reformulation of the first sentence in the definition of *vaccine* was no less than a clever piece of sleight of hand. It was immediately seized upon by pharma-friendly public health officials to persuade governments to impose mandatory treatments upon their citizens. Most political leaders have no formal training in science, and throughout their deliberations about what to do to address the COVID-19 outbreak, they were no doubt operating under the common assumptions that a *pandemic* is like the Black Plague, and a *vaccine* is a vaccine, in the sense of the 2018 definition. In fact, the redefinition of *vaccine* served a two-fold purpose: first, to rationalize universal vaccination programs and, second, to secure complete immunity for the product companies under the PREP Act.

Along with lawmakers, also hoodwinked, needless to say, was much of the populace, for many compliant citizens turned with great vigor and hatred against anyone who expressed "vaccine hesitancy." In fact, many of the "vaccine hesitant" were hesitant only to participate in an experimental trial for a novel mRNA treatment never before tested on human beings and which the product companies themselves claimed would moderate symptoms, not prevent transmission and infection.

There is no plausible way to understand these linguistic maneuvers other than as tactics deployed in order to promote any pharmaceutical product which those advising the government wish to sell. For the ability "to stimulate the body's immune response against diseases" is a very general and vague characteristic shared by many other substances not formerly categorized as vaccines at all. Using that definition, the government could force its citizenry to ingest a large number of products which may allay symptoms and make them less vulnerable to viruses but prevent neither infection nor transmission.

It stretches credulity to claim that somehow these definitions were arbitrarily or accidentally changed. Rather, the terms *pandemic* and *vaccine* were intentionally redefined precisely in order to promote a particular agenda, a program which will not be abandoned without ongoing and strenuous resistance by free people the world over. We have been warned and must remain vigilant against future attempts to usurp our bodily autonomy and freedom to conduct our lives as we see fit.

The U.S. legislation mounted during the Coronapocalypse, from the COVID Relief Acts to the Inflation Reduction Act, all deceptively suggested through their names that they would help the populace. In fact, they promoted, yet again, the interests of elites, precisely in the manner of the Ensuring Patient Access and Effective Drug Enforcement Act of 2014. What legislator could oppose bills with such titles? Only those who bother to read the texts of the legislation, which nearly none of the elected officials do. (Representative Thomas Massie stands out as a rare exception to the rule.) Instead, the alleged representatives of the people nearly always vote in concert with their Democratic or Republican colleagues, guided by enshrined senior legislators such as Nancy Pelosi and Mitch McConnell, who wield enormous power in directing funds to help or hinder the reelection of junior legislators. Even more importantly, figures such as Pelosi and McConnell are deeply indebted to the powerful lobbies in Washington, D.C., which donate generously only to lawmakers who promote the lobbyists' clients — above all, companies in the military and pharmaceutical industries.

A Government Ethos of Negligent Homicide

Whether or not one wishes to connect any further dots in the cases of drone assassination and the opioid epidemic, it does seem worth pointing out that Eric Holder, Obama's attorney general from 2009 to 2015, was a former legal counselor to Purdue Pharma, who in fact defended the company in a 2004 lawsuit alleging deceptive marketing of Oxycontin. This is noteworthy because it was none other than Eric Holder who, in an infamous White Paper and various public addresses, so adamantly defended the creative interpretation of *imminence* as not implying *immediacy*, the crucial linguistic maneuver used to defend and promote Obama's drone killing spree and his execution without trial or even indictment of U.S. citizens.

The normalization of assassination achieved by the Obama administration expanded the domain of what was said to be legitimate state killing by inverting the burden of proof on suspects while simultaneously claiming (illogically enough) that "areas outside active hostilities" were in fact war zones. Together, all of these linguistic tricks generated a veritable *killing machine*, opening up vast new market niches and dramatically increasing the profit potential for companies in the shockingly lucrative business of state-inflicted homicide. Not only weapons manufacturers but also logistics and analytics companies were able to reap hefty profits through eliminating as many people pegged as "terrorist suspects" as possible.

In a truly Orwellian move, the *imminent* vs. *immediate* dichotomy was inverted and redeployed, but in the opposite direction, by pharmaceutical company legal teams and collaborating lawmakers in 2014 to permit the promiscuous sale of narcotics to continue on despite the opioid overdose epidemic on display throughout the United States. The Ensuring Patient Access and Effective Drug Enforcement Act of 2014 ironically "ensured" only profits for drug companies, as millions of new addicts would be created during the second decade of the twenty-first century, accelerating and multiplying the domino effect of diversion and overdoses already ravaging communities all across the United States. It matters not that pharmaceutical company executives sought not to kill people but to sell pills. They aggressively pushed narcotics without regard for the likely future consequences of their drive for profit. Indeed, they persisted in pushing narcotics even as drug overdose deaths reached record levels.

In the "War on Terror" under Obama, more than 2,000 suspects outside areas of active hostilities were premeditatedly and intentionally incinerated by missiles launched from drones. The tally of overdose deaths in the United States exceeded 100,000 for the single year ending in April 2021. The long-range effects of the normalization of assassination, however, are likely to be more deadly than the opioid crisis, given that many other governments have followed suit[177] in acquiring lethal drones for their own use, having been persuaded by the precedent set by the U.S. government that this form of state-inflicted homicide is perfectly permissible.[178] In contrast, the promiscuous opioid prescription practices of doctors in the United States has been curtailed and was not emulated in the U.K. or in Europe, although the pharmaceutical giants do appear to have continued their morally dubious marketing practices in other countries abroad, especially in less-developed lands.

As the drone program normalization of assassination and the opioid prescription debacle already amply demonstrated, when government agencies such as the Pentagon and the FDA have been captured by industry forces focused above all on maximizing profits, they will simply look the other way as the corpses pile up, denying responsibility for any and all "collateral damage." No one should be surprised, then, that the handling of the COVID-19 crisis focused upon promoting pharmaceutical company interests even to the extreme extent that the manufacturing companies of the "vaccines" were granted complete immunity from lawsuits in the event of adverse effects on individual persons.

No one is held responsible in these cases, and the same old apology is offered to wipe the moral slate clean in matters of health as in matters of war: "We meant to do well." This by now permanent tendency of bureaucrats, elected officials, and corporate leaders to shirk responsibility for the negative consequences of their implemented policies helps to explain the ease with which lawmakers are coopted by lobbyists from not only the military but also the pharmaceutical industry. No one is held accountable, no matter what happens.

The twenty-first-century deployment of *imminent* and *immediate* by lethal legal "experts" in opposite directions serves to underscore why the censorship of language by government officials is inherently dangerous, given that their policies in recent years have multiplied, not prevented, the deaths of human beings. Likewise, without having redefined *pandemic* and *vaccine* so as to rationalize a massive upheaval of all of society and the transformation of citizens into frightened subjects, there could have been no grounds, even specious, for insisting on mandatory vaccine programs and health passports for what were formerly free people.

In a truly representative democracy, the lawmakers promote the interests of the voters who elected them. What kind of government sacrifices the lives of human beings in order to maximize the profits of corporate leaders?

20. The Smith-Mundt Modernization Act: From Propaganda to Censorship to Tyranny

May 18, 2022
Asheville, North Carolina

Spectacle and theater have come to dominate the political arena today, more so than ever before. Politicians are now celebrity oligarchs, who use tax revenues to promote their pet projects and to enhance their personal investment portfolios, while pretending in scrupulously orchestrated performances to care about the populace from whom all of the money they squander is siphoned. Congresspersons who issue dire warnings about global warming jet across the world for photo ops with President Zelensky in Ukraine. The provision by the federal government of Peloton bicycle memberships[179] to the House of Representatives and their staff, all on the taxpayer's dime, will begin on May 18, 2022. Meanwhile, more than 550,000 Americans are currently homeless. The absurdity of all of this has reached the point where we now seem to inhabit something akin to a sequel of *The Hunger Games.*

Consider the person recently selected by the Biden administration to head up its new Disinformation Governance Board (DGB), the self-styled "Mary Poppins of Disinformation,"[180] Nina Jankowicz, whose melodramatic mode of "correcting" what she takes to be falsehoods is disturbing to behold, to put it mildly. The DGB is being championed, needless to say, by spokespersons for President Biden, including former press secretary Jen Psaki,[181] who not only defended Jankowicz as "an expert on online disinformation" and "a person with extensive qualifications" but also expressed perplexity that anyone should take issue with the mounting of the DGB: "I'm not sure who opposes that effort."[182] This type of gaslighting should be recognized for what it is by now, for it has gone on throughout the Biden presidency, with officials responding with unbridled snark to anyone who raises perfectly valid questions about what they are doing. *How dare you?!*

"Our patience is wearing thin!" President Biden himself soberly warned the populace in denouncing the reluctance of some of his compatriots to volunteer as *pro bono* subjects in a Pfizer experimental medication trial. We were furthermore "informed" in December 2021 by the White House that, for our disobedience, we could look forward to "a winter of severe illness and death." Given the volume of such non-stop, and frankly surreal, psyops perpetrated on the populace since 2020, and before that as well — albeit usually more subtly — perhaps no one should have been surprised when a figure who could have been plucked directly from either *Hunger Games* or *Brazil* arrived on the scene to lead the charge against disinformation and "help" us to determine what we ought and ought not to believe. As if to test further the credulity and compliance of the populace (both of which were largely confirmed throughout the Coronapocalypse), the Biden administration selected to head up its dubious new board a person who has served as the functional equivalent of a Democratic Party operative for years.

Revulsion is a natural reaction to Jankowicz's appointment, but this particular piece of political theater strikes me as too "on the nose." The outcry on social media about "Mary Poppins" (whose performances have gone viral) is unlikely to subside anytime soon, which is why I surmise that the selection of Jankowicz may have been intended by the DGB masterminds as a red herring, to distract attention from the profound problems with the very idea of a Disinformation Governance Board. Perhaps the histrionic Jankowicz will be furloughed in response to a barrage of criticism from lawmakers on the right, to be replaced by a more staid and sober character, someone skilled at persuading television viewers that he speaks the truth. In that event, the U.S. populace and their ostensible representatives will have been duped.

Unfortunately, the victims of government-produced propaganda throughout the Coronapocalypse, which judging by its effects amounted to the psychological equivalent of a blunt-force head injury, have become more receptive than ever before to the latest propaganda lines and scams. "I got vaccinated" profile picture frames have been replaced with a beautiful Ukrainian flag, and some people are even donning t-shirts and displaying blue-and-yellow banners in their front yards alongside their "In this house we believe" rainbow placards. While lamenting inflation, caused directly by the profligate printing of currency by the government to fund COVID-19 "rescue" packages, those who support the latest print run of $40 billion for Ukraine appear to have been convinced by the government-vetted pundits on television (who else?) that, although Putin is incorrigibly evil and beyond the reach of reason, he would never, ever, even when repeatedly threatened with regime change and his personal demise, resort to the use of nuclear weapons, thus causing World War III and the end of human civilization.

Yes, after two years of government-inflicted trauma about a virus with a 99.5% survival rate, the cloth mask, mandatory vaxx crowd appear to have lost all critical bearings and stand ready to accept just about anything the government asks of them. The "Print $ for Ukraine" bill[183] includes massive allocations to the U.S. State Department ($14 billion), the U.S. Agency for International Development ($4.4 billion), and the Department of Defense ($20 billion) to dispense at their discretion, despite the government's pathetic record of failing to predict and thwart the terrorist attacks of 9/11, and its instigation since then of a variety of scandalous and immoral initiatives ranging from extraordinary rendition and torture to summary execution by lethal drones of suspects neither tried nor even indicted for crimes.

All of this mayhem got underway in the early twenty-first century with the government "apprising" citizens that Saddam Hussein had WMD (weapons of mass destruction) and was in cahoots with Osama bin Laden. Through such "intelligence community findings," citizens were deceived by "the experts" into believing that Iraq had something to do with 9/11 and therefore was fair game for attack in 2003. There can be little doubt that in the aftermath of the events of September 11, 2001, politicians' and the populace's critical faculties were compromised by the shock of what happened on that day, which best explains why they were so receptive to propaganda at the time.

Two decades later, George W. Bush, despite having wrecked much of the Middle East, now consults with and expresses enthusiastic support for Ukraine's President Zelensky, who is, according to Bush, "the Winston Churchill of our time." This farcical scenario serves above all to distract the discombobulated citizenry's attention from the fact that Bush's own invasion of Iraq bore similarities, not only to Putin's invasion of Ukraine, but also, yes, to Hitler's various military escapades. All of these leaders' campaigns were aggressive attacks on sovereign nations during peacetime.

How did we come to inhabit a society in which the government itself continually carries out psyops against the populace? There is a general sense in which the use of propaganda to manipulate the citizenry has always gone on — above all, during wartime — despite the fact that it undermines democracy by compromising the ability to ascertain the truth and to support policies *freely*, rather than being coerced through deception. A close examination of history (between the lines of textbooks written by spokespersons for the victors) reveals that the same sorts of mendacious tactics have been used by government officials and military leaders in their promotion and prolongation of most, if not all, wars. Fear is a powerful molder of minds, making citizens more, not less, receptive to leaders' lies.

When President Harry Truman spoke directly to U.S. citizens after the atomic bombing of Hiroshima in August 1945, he "informed" them that the target had been a military base. In reality, Hiroshima was a pristine site, never subjected to the firebombing suffered by dozens of other Japanese cities. That neither Hiroshima nor Nagasaki was bombed prior to being razed by Little Boy and Fat Man is best and indeed only explained by the fact that they were civilian, not military sites. But the horror of what was done to the residents of Hiroshima and Nagasaki is so shocking that, to this day, war supporters will go to extreme lengths to defend Truman's decision to destroy those cities. Bush administration officials went even so far as to contort the U.S. government's own use of atomic bombs into a rallying cry for war in 2003: "We don't want the smoking gun to be, a mushroom cloud!" We now know that Saddam Hussein had no WMD just as U.N. weapons inspector Hans Blix reported to the world before the Bush cabal waged war on Iraq anyway. Such examples illustrate that the distinction between "information" and "disinformation" purveyed by the government itself has always been difficult to discern in the moment of its utterance.

It is also true, however, that in 2013 President Barack Obama signed into law the Smith-Mundt Modernization Act (H.R. 5736), making it legal for government-produced media — such as was broadcast overseas by Voice of America, Radio Free Europe, and other outlets throughout the Cold War — to be directed toward U.S. citizens themselves. It goes without saying that such government-penned narratives spin the news so as to reflect favorably upon the United States. To understand the sheer power of the Smith-Mundt Modernization Act, it suffices to do a quick Google of the name of this piece of legislation to see how it has generated a logical quandary befitting of Orwell's *Nineteen Eighty-Four*. For if it is true that the American people are being propagandized by the U.S. government through its control of the major media outlets and tech giants, then any assertion to that effect will be countered — and ultimately defeated — by yet more government propaganda.

The fact that the complete negation of the original Smith-Mundt Act was deceptively labeled the Smith-Mundt *Modernization* Act[184] marked the first stage in what might be termed the Orwellian turn. Unsurprisingly, a lengthy list of articles calling out the alleged piece of "disinformation" that "Barack Obama legalized government propaganda against citizens" appears at the top of the Google search results. Among the critics who warned about the new Act was now-deceased investigative journalist Michael Hastings, who also, it is worth mentioning, expressed concern about the dangerous influence of the Pentagon's "public relations" wing, which already by 2009 employed 27,000 persons full-time as war marketeers.[185] A number of other notable figures who sounded alarms about the dangers of government propaganda and overreach are now dead, imprisoned, or living in exile.

The Smith-Mundt Modernization Act of 2012 (signed into law as a part of the National Defense Authorization Act of 2013) arguably set the United States on the path toward the erection of a full-fledged Ministry of Truth and the consequent shrinking of citizens' liberty. Only time will tell whether this piece of legislation alone will suffice, as deployed by the new Disinformation Governance Board, to strip citizens of their First Amendment right to free speech when they attempt to reject the first premises of the DGB itself. If so, then Barack Obama will bear primary responsibility for the totalitarian system to ensue, whatever his intentions may have been.

For with the Smith-Mundt Modernization Act already in place, there are only two short steps to the complete squelching of dissent. First, the government controls the media through injecting many pro-government texts into the marketplace of ideas. This is obviously already being done, and has been unabashedly pursued since the ratification of the Act. (To dispel any doubts that this is happening, it suffices to turn on the mainstream network news.) Second, among the government-promoted ideas will now be the claim that the newly established Disinformation Governance Board does not violate the Constitution of the United States. Once lawmakers have been persuaded to believe this, then the DGB will have the power to eliminate what they themselves have identified as disinformation, including the very claim that the DGB is illegitimate. After that will follow the censorship of the texts of anyone who disagrees with the government and, ultimately, the criminalization of those who "persist" in promulgating ideas deemed "threatening" by the powers that be. The danger of all of this to free people is very real, as the plight of whistleblowers in recent years has already revealed.

The very claim that any human being is "qualified" to serve as the Czar of Truth illustrates how ignorant the supporters of this frightening initiative are of the history of censorship used by dictators to eliminate inconvenient opinions — that is, those which conflict with the current group of administrators' policies and beliefs. It also helps to explain what happened from 2020 to 2022, when a single man, Anthony Fauci, was decreed by the U.S. government the final authority on "The Science" and transformed into the darling of the mainstream media.

The first generation of pandemic propagandists studied and deployed the fear-based post-9/11 playbook. (Given the impressive profits reaped by Pfizer,[186] there will likely be more, especially since the word *pandemic* has been redefined to encompass such illnesses as the flu and the common cold.) In 2020, when citizens were "informed" by public health guru Anthony Fauci and vaccine entrepreneur Bill Gates that they were facing something akin to the Black Plague, necessitating that they cease all social activity and refuse to leave their homes, nearly everyone fell in line. Lockdowns, mandatory vaccinations, schoolchildren forced to wear masks and either Zoom from home or work at desks enclosed by Plexiglas — all of this was just part of "the new normal" with which many citizens were willing to comply, in heartfelt efforts to save their own and their loved ones' lives.

Throughout 2020 and 2021, government officials and their associated mainstream media pundits "informed us" that citizens are not capable of doing their own research. That doctors who disagreed with public health officials were quacks. That unpatented treatments were so ineffective (and poisonous!) that the government needed to ban them. Looking back over all that has transpired, it seems difficult to deny that the notion that only pro-Big Pharma supporters are qualified to give sound medical advice was just another Pfizer-sponsored marketing line — not at all unlike the FDA-approved propaganda used to persuade, and indeed pressure, doctors to prescribe and patients to ingest powerful narcotics marketed as nonaddictive, when in fact they directly generated the opioid crisis raging on still today.

Among other recently debunked disinformation disseminated by the government, we know that the Hunter Biden laptop was neither planted by the Russians nor a "Trump campaign product," as Ms. Jankowicz herself so confidently (and cleverly!) characterized it in October 2020.[187] The supposed appointment by the Russian government of Donald Trump as president also never took place, *pace* Hillary Clinton, who, it seems safe to say, will go to her grave championing that now-debunked tale. Holding a master's degree in "disinformation studies" from Georgetown University makes Jankowicz as qualified as anyone else to be the Czar of Truth. But that's only because no human being is or ever could be qualified to hold such a position.

Any head of the DGB (whether Jankowicz or her Republican Party-approved replacement) will represent an administration which vociferously promoted the use of cloth masks, pushed for mandatory vaccinations, ignored the reality of natural immunity, and claimed that the Hunter Biden laptop was planted by the Russians. The path forward, therefore, seems clear. All we need to do, given the government's easily documented record of promoting manifest falsehoods, is to adopt a simple heuristic device. We should conclude *not-p* whenever the head of the DGB asserts that *p* is the truth. When the claim is made (as it will continue to be) that "The Deep State does not exist," we should conclude that it does. When the Czar of Truth asserts that 2 + 2 = 5, we should obviously conclude that it is not the case that 2 + 2 = 5.

To take the most pressing of current examples, we have good grounds for believing that the government's position on the Ukraine-Russia conflict is precisely the opposite of the truth. Indeed, the very fact that confirmed war criminal George W. Bush[188] has taken time out of his portrait painting schedule to promote the proxy war against Russia should bolster our belief. Yes, the same George W. Bush who triumphantly announced the end of his Iraq war on May 1, 2003, during a superlative theatrical performance on the deck/stage of an aircraft carrier where he wore as his costume a fighter pilot's jacket and stood before a huge banner proclaiming *Mission Accomplished!*

Through concerted campaigns of fearmongering, citizens have been reduced over the course of the twenty-first century to the intellectual equivalent of small children who helplessly accept whatever "the adults" decree and parrot precepts such as that we must leave all weighty matters to "the experts" — as though the persons in appointed positions were not specially selected by politicians with agendas to promote and stock portfolios to enrich. Those who wave their Ukrainian flags continue to labor under a barrage of government-generated propaganda and seem to have forgotten already that the wealthiest military on the planet was unable to prevail against the ragtag Taliban in Afghanistan. The bulk of voters derive all of their information about foreign policy from the government-captured mainstream media and tech giants. (Yemen? Where's Yemen? Who cares?) As a result, most people appear to be altogether oblivious to the magnitude of corruption uncovered by audits of the taxpayer funds dispensed throughout the Global War on Terror.

Supporters of the proxy war in Ukraine express moral indignation that Senator Rand Paul should have delayed the doling out of billions of freshly printed money "for Ukraine" by insisting that an Inspector General report back on how the funds are spent. But the truth is the truth, no matter what the government's propaganda ministry may say. After spending trillions of dollars on the "War on Terror," enriching mercenaries and war profiteers all along the way, while slaying hundreds of thousands of innocent people and wrecking the lives of many more, Afghanistan was left to the Taliban, who naturally inherited all of the wartime *matériel* left behind by the invaders of their land.

As anyone familiar with intellectual history is well aware, the problem posed by the DGB is not peculiar to the current crop of corrupt and coopted hypocrites holding positions in the U.S. government. In order for any committee headed up by anyone anywhere to be able to pronounce authoritatively whether a given utterance is a piece of disinformation or not, they would need to have some means for distinguishing truth from mere opinion, and knowledge from mere belief. The perennial philosophical problem, addressed by thinkers at least as far back as Socrates and Plato, is that human beings are inextricably mired in opinion and belief. In creating democratic societies, modern people rejected Plato's notion of *Philosopher Kings*, who, having made their way out of *The Cave*, supposedly have privileged access to *The Truth*. In recognition of the fallibility and limited perspectives of all human beings, Western liberal states have affirmed, through their constitutions, the importance of John Stuart Mill's marketplace of ideas. Accordingly, they have devised mechanisms, courts of law, by which to resolve disagreements over the facts.

That the newly created Disinformation Governance Board should have been announced at about the same time as the leak of what looks to be the impending *Roe v. Wade* reversal by the U.S. Supreme Court may or may not be coincidental. But the peril of permitting government appointees to decree from their position what is and is not disinformation, while simultaneously undermining the legitimacy of the court system, cannot be exaggerated.

Without the court system, as flawed as it is and can only be, since all parties involved are fallible human beings, we would find ourselves in the sorry system of not just our current corrupt oligarchy but a full-fledged tyranny disguised as a democracy.

The danger before us is not, however, merely domestic. Despite all that we have been through and learned about the sheer incompetence of public health and other government officials over the course of the twenty-first century, the WHO is maneuvering to establish a global governance scheme which will strip from all citizens of participating nations their civil rights in the event of the arrival of another pandemic on the scene. Now that *pandemic* has been redefined by "the experts" to include viruses such as COVID-19 with a 99.5% survival rate (similar to that of the seasonal flu), such a treaty would spell the end of personal liberty and bodily autonomy, with citizens criminalized for not accepting injections of whatever the WHO deems necessary in the name of public health. If this initiative succeeds, it will be because politicians, who are no less vulnerable to propaganda than anyone else, have been persuaded to accede to a treaty which effectively enslaves their constituents.

21. A COVID Coda

August 30, 2022
Tucson, Arizona

Anthony Fauci has announced that he will step down from his position as director of the National Institute of Allergy and Infectious Diseases (NIAID) and, more importantly for free people, his role as the *de facto* public health czar of the United States. He has indicated that he is not retiring but moving on to the next chapter of his career, which I surmise will involve serving as Global Health Guru to the World Health Organization (WHO) or perhaps even the World Economic Forum (WEF).

Since the spring of 2020, through a non-stop mainstream media campaign, Fauci succeeded in persuading U.S. politicians all across the country — at the federal, state, and local level — to implement arbitrary, ineffectual policies supposedly designed by experts to protect the small portion of the population vulnerable to COVID-19, policies which spelled disaster and even death for thousands of others.

Despite having spent a greater percentage of its GDP in response to COVID-19 than any other country on the planet except Singapore,[189] the United States had the worst outcome among all wealthy nations, not only in terms of virus victim deaths per capita, but also in excess mortality (non-virus deaths), which was the direct result of government policies.[190] Fauci & Co. also pushed an experimental mRNA treatment on pregnant women (who had been excluded from the initial pharmaceutical company trials) and children, for whom dying from COVID-19 is far less likely than is accidental death.[191]

Supporters of Fauci will brush the statistics aside, charitably observing that "to err is human," but his willingness actively to suppress any dissent in the name of public health uniquely qualifies him to lead the charge to strip people worldwide of bodily autonomy and the freedom to dissent, both of which appear to be key planks in the Great Global Reset. I could be wrong. It may be that Tony is just going to sail off into the sunset on his Pfizer, Moderna, and Johnson & Johnson laurels, securing an even more lucrative consulting gig with one of the companies whose CEOs became a billionaire overnight[192] thanks to the government's corporate welfare programs disguised as public health. No, the "vaccines" were not free. Were they even vaccines?

In fact, the mRNA shot was always a one-trick pony, designed only to galvanize the body to produce a foreign spike protein (used by the original virus to gain access to cells), which would then elicit a robust antibody response. It is through mutation that viruses manage to propagate themselves in hostile environments. In this case, what was needed for survival was to evade the spike protein antibodies and find new ways to gain entry into the cells of potential hosts. Accordingly, given the rate of virus mutation in general, the original strain may not even exist anymore.[193] Yet the products administered to patients since 2021, long past their "best before" date, have been rebranded as "boosters." The formula of the shots is the same, but the virus has undergone significant mutation specifically to render nugatory the antibodies produced in response to injection of the spike protein mRNA.

All of that said, if people are still interested in increasing the amount of spike protein in their system, it remains their prerogative to roll up their sleeve. Your body, your choice. I ask only that the Faucistas (who obviously never read *The Real Anthony Fauci* by Robert F. Kennedy, Jr., or any book on Big Pharma, for that matter) simply leave me alone. Yes, it's been a long two and a half years, and I am frankly tired of trying to reason with people who want so ardently to believe, that they will never read any article, much less an entire book, critical of the Fauci-CNN narrative. They will no doubt continue to cling to the saving grace afforded to "America's Doctor"[194] by "Causation or correlation?" as they deny that anyone could possibly be responsible for any of the harm done.

The elderly grandparents who died in isolation, unable to hug their loved ones goodbye; the small children prevented from socializing normally during the formative years of their development; the many patients who missed their cancer screenings and will as a result die earlier than they might have; the marked increase in suicides and drug overdoses among persons financially and psychologically ruined by the lockdowns. And let us not downplay the enduring and divisive ugliness which drove people to cease interacting with friends and family members who refused to undergo an experimental treatment offering them very little (~1%) risk reduction and which *did not stop transmission anyway.*[195]

Many of the public figures who insisted that vaccination would prevent infection have now had COVID-19, in some cases, multiple times. That should settle the matter once and for all, and yet there are still mandates in place for military personnel and others who continue to be coerced into undergoing experimental medical procedures in direct violation of the Nuremberg Code (see Appendix B). Despite the irrefutable proof that the shots prevent neither transmission nor infection, as demonstrated by the multiple infections of the quadruply-jabbed President Joe Biden and First Lady Jill Biden, the mayor of Washington, D.C., Muriel Bowser, recently decreed that children will not be allowed in public school classrooms this fall[196] without first undergoing an experimental medical treatment of which they have no need.

The already shrinking middle class was hit especially hard by the politically engineered response to the COVID-19 crisis, which effected the largest transfer of wealth in history from the thousands of small businesses destroyed to a handful of megacorporations which were up and running all along, having been designated "essential." The purchase by the government of millions of shots — labeled for marketing purposes "vaccines" — to be universally administered to citizens, who in some countries were then required to take them on pain of severe penalties for refusal to do so, was another enormous transfer of wealth, in this case, to Big Pharma.

Much to the chagrin of the young people who developed myocarditis subsequent to injection,[197] the companies which produced the shots were granted blanket immunity in the event of adverse effects, even as people were coerced into taking them by threats of job loss and exclusion from travel, school, and participation in society. To this day, no foreign visitor is allowed to enter the United States without proof of vaccination.[198] In some ways even more devastating (to anyone but Big Pharma grifters and profiteers) has been the creation of a not-insignificant number of hypochondriacs who continue to conduct themselves as though contact with other people is likely to be fatal.

The CDC recently issued a long overdue statement affirming some of the core tenets of the Great Barrington Declaration of October 4, 2020 (see Appendix A), which you may recall led to a vicious campaign of discreditation and deplatforming of anyone who dared to disagree with Anthony "The Science" Fauci.[199] Among other things, the CDC has now finally acknowledged that persons previously infected with COVID-19 do have protection, a claim which was either overtly or tacitly denied throughout the lengthy initial vaccine-marketing period, when President Biden oscillated between attempting to persuade and denouncing as deplorable those who continued to decline the vaccines.

Those of us who dared to believe in what were considered up until March 2020 veritable truisms of immunology — first and foremost, that because we had already recovered, we did not need to roll up our sleeves — were subjected to an endless barrage of harassment and restrictions, on top of being spurned as pariahs by fellow citizens (and even family members!) who had been assiduously indoctrinated by our very own government to believe that we were selfish, evil people. Leading the charge of the torch-wielding mandate mob, the White House solemnly intoned around Christmastime 2021 that justice would prevail, as we would be punished for our disobedience with a "winter of severe illness and death." Alas (to those who reviled anyone who refused to comply, no matter the reason), most of the unwashed, unvaxxed, unmasked masses survived.

A second previously received wisdom, that genuine vaccines prevent infection and transmission, was overturned through fiat, by redefining the term *vaccine* so as to make it possible to label the COVID-19 mRNA spike protein shot as such in order to maximize sales and, indeed, to serve as the pretext for universal mandates to be imposed by governments. Over the course of the Coronapocalypse, many public figures have broadcast their positive COVID-19 test as some sort of mark of their fortitude, invariably accompanied by a heartfelt expression of gratitude for the fact that they were vaccinated, as a result of which their symptoms were mild. People with access to the auxiliary Pfizer product, Paxlovid,[200] have also gushed about how they are recovering thanks only to Pfizer.

It is a preposterous conceit to claim that Pfizer saved the life of anyone who was in nearly no danger of losing it, as was always the case for infected persons neither already plagued by comorbidities nor extremely old and frail. People in those cohorts are also the ones who tend to die of the flu, although there are rare cases where young healthy people do as well. But let's all just credit Pfizer with our ongoing existence, because, well, we are still alive!

Compounding this fraud is that the Pfizer shots were paid for by the U.S. government twice: through the infusion of massive funding for research and production, and then the subsequent purchase of the individual doses and attempted mandates of their use. Yes, acting as the most effective of all possible marketers, the government attempted to coerce us into taking the shots, even when we knew from published scientific literature (not authored by Fauci) as early as April 2021[201] that our personal risk reduction of less than 1% would have to be weighed against an unknown probability of long-term adverse vaccine side effects. The products were fast-tracked to receive Emergency Use Authorization, and the experimental trials were not set to end until 2023, according to the manufacturers' own fact sheets.

"Mistakes were made" does not even begin to address how what appears to have been a virus engineered through gain-of-function research brought back by none other than Anthony Fauci himself caused the deaths of millions of human beings all over the world.[202] But even setting that concern to one side, even if, against the overwhelming genome-sequencing evidence,[203] the virus leapt naturally from bats to homo sapiens when someone in Wuhan ate a bowl of soup, the toll of destruction left in Fauci's wake is nonetheless damning.

For it was Fauci's instituted protocol that persons with mild symptoms be sent home until they were sick enough to require ventilators. It was Fauci's prescription that the toxic[204] and ineffective[205] antiviral drug Remdesivir be administered to thousands of ailing patients, many of whom ended up dying. It was Fauci who ridiculed attempts by "rogue" medical doctors to save their patients' lives through early and preemptive treatments with therapeutics which might cut into the profits of the vaccine makers. All of this is criminal, and it will not be ignored by the future historians who assess what really went on during this period of government-induced mass hysteria.

In the aftermath of the disastrous political handling of the COVID-19 virus, which, if not literally created through government-funded gain-of-function research, was in any case turned into a crisis by the government, the middle class continues to be hollowed out as regular, working people are pushed to penury by rising prices, rents, and taxes, in some cases finally losing the roof over their heads. At present, there are an estimated 600,000 homeless Americans, and more than 100,000 persons died of drug overdoses over the course of the past year.[206] The overdose epidemic did not begin with COVID-19 but was made worse by the loss of meaningful activities, as people forbidden from working in some cases supplemented their Netflix and pizza binges with readily available fentanyl-laced drugs of unknown provenance.[207]

Critical thinkers should by now be well aware that the printing of money by a central government authority can only exacerbate inflation. But the sad story of how the opioid overdose epidemic itself began, the role played by the FDA (Food and Drug Administration) in helping to promote the use of supposedly "nonaddictive narcotics," appears to be less widely recognized.[208] Never fear, Compliant and Gullible Citizens, to a range of government-created problems, we have to the rescue once again… (drum roll)… the government!

The Orwellian "Inflation Reduction Act" recently signed into U.S. law[209] provides for the hiring of 87,000 new IRS agents whose job requirements include the willingness to bear arms and to use deadly force, "when necessary." (Because failure to pay taxes is now a capital offense?) Note that the "Assault Weapons Ban" (H.R. 1808)[210] passed by the House of Representatives to restrict citizens' access to weapons such as the AR-15 provides an explicit exception for "law enforcement officers," presumably to include the ones who will soon be showing up on the doorsteps of businesses and individuals believed by the government to have evaded federal tax law.

Given that large corporations are all protected by armies of lawyers, it seems likely that the main targets of this hunt for new funds will be small businesses, ironically, those robust enough to have survived what amounted to the COVID-19 lockdown purge. I would be surprised if it were not the case that among the survivors were indeed some who fudged their numbers here and there, which means that we should in the not-too-distant future see even more small businesses disappear.

As a simple example of what was probably illegal but fully comprehensible tax evasion, as no doubt occurred all over the world given the dire circumstances created by lockdowns, I recall my experience in Surrey (U.K.) in October 2020, when I enlisted the services of a taxi driver to transport me to the train station. He adamantly refused to accept as payment anything but cash, offering even to take me to an ATM, if need be. I assumed at the time that the fellow must have been struggling to survive, even to keep a roof over his head, given the drastic reduction in movement of people caused by the government's restrictions and, consequently, the radically diminished need for his services. Meanwhile, politicians who were never in any danger of losing their means of sustenance doled out billions of dollars of nonexistent funds to implement their feckless and myopic policies by effectively printing money to be paid for by future generations (see the Debt Clock[211]).

Alas, in these Tertullian times, the more preposterous the logic, the more irresistible it becomes. It cannot be that all of society was shut down for a virus with a 99.5% survival rate. So it must be the case that, if the government had not done what it did, then the outcome would have been much, much worse. That's the marketing line which has been successfully insinuated into the minds of millions of people who continue to credit their ongoing existence to a "vaccine" which prevents neither infection nor transmission and offers very little risk reduction to healthy persons devoid of the sorts of comorbidities which attended nearly all COVID-19 deaths. These people have been duped into believing that the government is their savior, and they will comply with whatever is said to be necessary for the common good. The alternative — that they have been not only robbed but also psychologically traumatized by elected officials and their appointees — is simply too awful to embrace. Accordingly, they can be expected to continue to light their votive candles to Saint Fauci, regardless of the body count he left in his wake.

22. Happy New Year: The Government Did Not Save Your Life

January 9, 2023
Salt Lake City, Utah

More than 100,000 persons died of narcotics overdoses last year in the United States, in many cases because the street drugs they used were laced with extremely potent fentanyl. If you were among the survivors of a dose of unknown provenance, the reason you are alive is that you were lucky. If the government had not made it illegal to purchase and sell drugs, then people would not have to resort to shady dealers in dark alleys and literally gamble their lives away when they ingested such substances.

Not all victims of fentanyl overdose have been drug addicts, but some of them were, and in order to obtain their needed fix, they were driven to acquire narcotics by all means necessary. Many of them became that way because they trusted their doctors, who trusted the government's Food and Drug Administration (FDA). If you were prescribed narcotics for minor bouts of pain during the early years of what became the opioid crisis and overdose epidemic, and you did not become addicted to your pills, that is not because but in spite of the government.

You prudently declined to empty your large amber vial, knowing as you did, as have the people of many societies for centuries, that narcotics are in fact highly addictive. You did not believe the marketing hype condoned by the FDA, according to which powerful narcotics had suddenly become nonaddictive. Far from being protected by the government, the victims of the opioid crisis were sacrificed on the altar of Big Pharma because their cronies in government permitted them to convince doctors and patients alike that their new wonder drugs were safe and could and should be liberally ingested by anyone for virtually anything. Doctors not only trusted but were also pressured by the pharma-coopted federal regulatory agencies to prescribe the patented pills. Patients believed what their doctors told them, and the rest is history.[212]

Thousands of persons in the United States died of respiratory illnesses in 2022, as they do each year. Many of them had been inoculated, in some cases quadruply, with the elixir persistently promoted by the government as the solution to the COVID-19 pandemic, even as rapidly mutating variants rendered the original shots nugatory. Although the substance injected into human bodies billions of times from 2021 to 2022 was labeled a *vaccine*, in reality, deaths from the virus which it was designed to combat increased rather than decreased in the period following widespread inoculation campaigns in countries all over the world.

If you survived COVID-19, then unless you are elderly, obese, or beset with multiple comorbidities, the government did not save your life. (And if you did fall into those categories and were exposed to the virus as a result of "public health" officials' guidance to political leaders such as Governor Cuomo in New York to send infected persons to convalesce in nursing homes, then you might well number among the people not reading these words because they will never read any words ever again.) In truth, you are alive because you were never vulnerable to the "severe illness and death" by COVID-19 used in the ubiquitous marketing campaign to persuade you to volunteer as a subject in the largest experimental trial of a medical devicc (the novel mRNA technology) in history.

If you are not one of the thousands of formerly healthy persons who have dropped dead from cardiac arrest or a blood clot-induced stroke since being coerced by your employer, under pressure by the government, to accept a medical treatment of which you had no need, the government certainly did not save your life. The mounting evidence suggests that the causal factor in these "unexplained" cases was the biologically active spike protein created by bodies injected with the mRNA coding for the production of that foreign substance. Many people succumbed to the overwhelming pressure put upon them to undergo an unnecessary treatment, up to and including the threat of the abrupt ending of their career. But according to all available statistical data, healthy persons under the age of seventy were always unlikely (<0.5%) to die from COVID-19, whether with or without treatment. If you number among that cohort and opted for "vaccination," then you are in all likelihood alive today because your body did not overproduce the biologically active spike protein coded for by the mRNA injected into your arm — the same spike protein used by the COVID-19 virus to penetrate cells. Your body did not keep producing that potentially harmful substance, and it did not coalesce within any of your organ systems. There is no sense in which the government saved your life by persuading or coercing you to undergo an experimental treatment of which you had no need. Rather, you just got lucky that your body happened to produce foreign-coded protein inefficiently. Or perhaps your dose was weak or expired.

Homeless people die every winter in cities such as New York, Chicago, Philadelphia, Salt Lake City, and Denver, to name but a few. If you are alive today, in 2023, it is not because the government saved your life. It is because you were fortunate enough not to have been sabotaged by the lockdowns which prevented healthy persons in the gig economy from earning enough money to pay for adequate shelter. Some among the homeless victims have succumbed to drug use and suffered overdose deaths.[213] The fact that you had a salaried position during the Coronapocalypse, and were thus able to weather the politically generated storm, has nothing to do with the government — unless, of course, you happen to be a government employee… Either way, you simply numbered among the lucky.

Not all of the homeless persons in the United States are veterans of the wars of vanity, choice, and greed instigated by the military industry-coopted government in the twenty-first century, but some of them are. Beyond the military veterans who succumb to the elements or suffer overdose deaths, thousands more take their lives each year. They have been psychologically destroyed by their experiences fighting in dubious wars where they are ordered to kill or witness the killing of people who manifestly do not deserve to die. If you are alive today, it is not because the government saved your life by sacrificing so many enlisted men and women, or by killing, maiming, and terrorizing millions of innocent persons abroad. It is because you were lucky enough neither to be hoodwinked by wartime recruitment propaganda nor to need to sign your life away in order to be able to support yourself and your family or to pay for your education.

If you did not starve to death in 2022, it's not because the government saved your life. Thank your lucky stars that you were not born in Yemen, where a brutal U.S.-supported war has been raging on between the Saudis and the Houthis since 2015. Through initiating and perpetuating this conflict, the U.S. government has not made you any safer, whether by arming the Saudis in their ruthless slaughter, or by facilitating their savage blockades. Instead, the government has helped to sow misery and death throughout that land, as a direct result of which hundreds of thousands of innocent people have perished, not only in the crossfire of the military conflict, but also from starvation and disease.

If you were not vaporized in a nuclear holocaust in 2022, it's not because your government saved your life. It's because Russian President Vladimir Putin, armed to the teeth with nuclear weapons inherited by Russia from the U.S.S.R., has not yet succumbed to the threats of regime change and imminent personal demise incessantly pumped out by U.S. "statesmen." Rather than facilitate the negotiated ending of what is effectively a dispute between Russia and Ukraine over a border established three decades ago by a small committee of men, the U.S. government has pumped enormous amounts of money and arms into the region, more than $100 billion to date, a sum in excess of the entire military budget of Russia. Through serially threatening Putin, representatives of the U.S. government have in no way protected you. Instead, they have relentlessly and recklessly whittled away at the first premises of the theory of Mutually Assured Destruction (MAD).

According to MAD, developed during the Cold War, back when the Soviet Union still existed and posed a real threat to free people, neither party to a conflict between two nuclear powers will resort to the use of such weapons of mass annihilation, provided that they believe that their side will suffer unacceptable losses in the triggered ricochet effect initiated by the first strike. But if a leader with his finger on the button of nuclear weapons comes to believe as a result of credible threats that he is on the verge of being assassinated, then all bets are off. Any government which continually provokes the leader of a nuclear-armed nation to believe that he is going to be "taken out" by them is either ignorant of, or disregards the basis for, MAD.

The sabotage of the Nord Stream pipelines on September 26, 2022, remains a yet-to-be-solved mystery, even though before it happened U.S. officials rendered themselves the most likely suspects by publicly proclaiming that, if Russia invaded Ukraine, then the pipelines would not go forward.[214] If in fact that crime was committed by the U.S. government, which would make it tantamount to a declaration of war, and Putin believes this to be the case, knowing as he does better than anyone else that Russia did not sabotage its own project, then your ongoing existence rests, again, only on the restraint exhibited by the Russian president in refraining to retaliate against the perpetrators of the sabotage.

The fact that Putin has not opted to use nuclear weapons, given that he has been repeatedly informed/threatened by U.S. leaders that he will be removed from power, by hook or by crook, may ironically enough be a result of the fact that the U.S. government no longer has any credibility on foreign policy.[215] Whatever the reason that Putin has declined up to now to use all of the tools at his disposal, rest assured that you are not alive because your government saved your life. Instead, you lucked out that Putin happens not to be as impulsive as U.S. warmakers, who assassinate anyone they want, anywhere they want, in a complete state of impunity, and appear fully prepared to plot Putin's demise as well, civilization be damned. As though oblivious to why and how all of humanity was not wiped out in a nuclear conflagration during the Cold War, representatives of the U.S. government persist in provoking Putin to the point of wondering whether his assassination is on the CIA's list of things to make and do. Lucky for you, Putin does not yet believe them.

Of course, if there were no nuclear weapons, then no leader of any government would be in the position to destroy millions of human beings with the push of a button. Weapons powerful enough to wipe out large swaths of humanity were developed in the MAD arms race over the course of the decades-long U.S.-U.S.S.R. conflict, as the Soviet Union endeavored not only to expand but also to protect itself through nuclear deterrence. If the U.S. government had never developed atomic bombs and demonstrated its willingness to use them by dropping them on the civilian cities of Hiroshima and Nagasaki in 1945, then the nuclear arms race between the Soviet Union and the United States would likely not have taken place. The government's production of weapons of mass destruction has not enhanced but undermined your security. If you are old enough to have lived through the Cold War, then the fact that you happened to survive was an extraordinary stroke of luck, as we know from multiple close calls, the most famous of which was the Cuban Missile Crisis.

23. The Meaning of the COVID-19 Vaccine Mandates in 2023

January 17, 2023
Holladay, Utah

On September 18, 2022, President Joe Biden told a CBS news reporter in a *60 Minutes* interview that "the pandemic is over."[216] Two months later, on November 16, 2022, at a G20 meeting in Bali, Biden signed, on behalf of the United States, a declaration which states (in Article 19) that "the pandemic is not over." Among the provisions of the lengthy G20 agreement[217] is a green light for the possibility of a legally binding global (supranational) vaccination passport scheme, ostensibly to facilitate international travel:

> We support the work of the Intergovernmental Negotiating Body (INB) that will draft and negotiate a legally binding instrument that should contain both legally binding and non-legally binding elements to strengthen pandemic PPR and the working group on the International Health Regulations that will consider amendments to the International Health Regulations (IHR) (2005) mindful that the decision will be made by World Health Assembly.
> (Article 19)

> We acknowledge the importance of shared technical standards and verification methods, under the framework of the IHR (2005), to facilitate seamless international travel, interoperability, and recognizing digital solutions and non-digital solutions, including proof of vaccinations. We support continued international dialogue and collaboration on the establishment of trusted global digital health networks as part of the efforts to strengthen prevention and response to future pandemics, that should capitalize and build on the success of the existing standards and digital COVID-19 certificates.
> (Article 23)

By the end of 2022, three months after Biden's claim that the pandemic had ended, the United States was still requiring non-citizens to present proof of vaccination at the border — a requirement imposed only by these other countries as of today: Azerbaijan, Indonesia, Myanmar, and Pakistan. This despite the fact that the president himself (quadruply-jabbed at that time) had already been infected with COVID-19, thus demonstrating for all the world that the shots did not stop the spread of the virus.[218]

While Biden was busy abroad networking with globalist friends whose plans have far-reaching, indeed universal effects, a few members of the U.S.

Congress, including Representative Thomas Massie of Kentucky, were working diligently in the homeland on legislation to repeal the COVID-19 vaccine mandate on military personnel. As Massie and many others have repeatedly (and cogently) observed, a so-called vaccine which does not prevent infection and transmission serves no public health purpose whatsoever, and a mandate on groups, including large groups such as the military, does not protect the members of the group from the possibility of infection by other members of the group. Without what has proven to be a spurious public health pretext, promoted through an aggressive, relentless propaganda campaign, the decision of whether or not to undergo inoculation can only remain, rationally speaking, a private medical choice for individuals to make for themselves in consultation with their doctors.

The military imposes a variety of medical requirements upon troops in the name of battlefield readiness, but mandating a medical treatment for the military corps in this case was especially dubious, for one of the well-documented side effects of the experimental mRNA shots is myocarditis, and this ailment, while rare, is most common among younger males. Requiring healthy young men at nearly no risk of death from the COVID-19 virus itself to undergo a treatment which has as a possible side effect organ injury, or even death, makes no sense whatsoever, except perhaps as a policy of forced submission. Yes, a soldier is duty-bound to follow orders. But the reason for that is supposed to be related to the importance of coordination in potentially dangerous operations, where a failure to follow orders may result in the deaths of the soldier's comrades and ultimately jeopardize not only the mission but also the greater battle underway.

The Biden administration's COVID-19 "vaccine" mandate on soldiers had the opposite effect of the presumed requirement of obedience. Rather than increasing the battlefield readiness of the military corps, about 8,400 enlisted persons were relieved (without pay) of their positions for refusing to follow the dubious order. It is perhaps worth pointing out here that the loss of this particular subset of the larger group arguably constituted, at the same time, something of a brain drain on the military, leaving behind a less intelligent group, given that the persons forbidden from serving had refused to submit mindlessly to what was manifestly an illogical order.

A more complicated moral argument could be made here as well. If we accept the Nuremberg court findings, then the requirement of obedience does not absolve a soldier in all cases from culpability in having followed illegal orders.[219] If a human being has a right not to be experimented on against his will, as the Nuremberg Code (see Appendix B) itself affirms, then in refusing to accede to such an order, the soldier is in fact complying with the court's broader ruling on obedience, although in the case of the mRNA shots, the person not to be violated is the soldier himself. Pentagon officials maintain, of course, that the order to undergo vaccination was legal, having evidently failed to comprehend the inherent contradiction (or simple Newspeak) of a "vaccine" which prevents neither infection nor transmission.

The shot may serve a therapeutic purpose, by making infection less severe and deadly to persons *already* vulnerable to those outcomes (because they are elderly, infirm, and/or obese), but for the vast majority of persons in the active military, who are young and healthy, the risk reduction of the shots is minimal, indeed less than 1%, whichever of the various shots one considers. A consciously inculcated equivocation between Absolute Risk Reduction (ARR) and Relative Risk Reduction (RRR) began with the very launch of the vaccines, the resplendent projected success of which was based upon analysis of likely outcomes in *vulnerable* cohorts, not among the young and healthy persons who comprise much of the military corps.[220]

In the end, the argument made by the Republican congresspersons who succeeded in halting the military's COVID-19 vaccine mandate had nothing whatsoever to do with the fact that the shots may harm young people, nor that any rational risk-benefit analysis would side with the troops who declined to roll up their sleeves, given that they are among the least vulnerable of all cohorts to the virus itself, and the shots do not prevent infection and transmission anyway. The primary line of reasoning used to persuade Congress to outlaw the mandate (and pressed by Republican governors[221] as well) made no mention of the Nuremberg Code, human rights, or bodily autonomy — specifically the right of free persons to decide which substances to introduce into their very own bodies. Instead, lawmakers maintained that by reducing the number of active-duty troops, the mandate was jeopardizing national security.

The history of the military's use of soldiers as subjects in a variety of experiments, often without their knowledge, much less informed consent, reveals a notoriously cavalier attitude among administrators toward exposing soldiers to toxic substances such as Agent Orange in Vietnam, the emanations of bombed chemical factories during Operation Desert Storm (the 1991 Gulf War), and the burn pit fumes in Afghanistan and Iraq in the twenty-first-century "War on Terror." Given the persistence with which injured soldiers' claims have been diminished or outright denied by authorities in conflict after conflict, it seems fairly clear that, from the perspective of the military's top brass, a soldier's right to bodily autonomy is effectively renounced upon enlistment. The implicit logic, reduced to its essence, seems to be something like this: if a person is already willing to sacrifice his life for his country, then every lesser sacrifice may be asked of him as well.

The relatively recent acknowledgement by the Biden administration of the damage caused to soldiers by the burn pits may be attributable to the fact that President Biden believes that his own son Beau was one of the victims, having developed brain cancer and died as a result of exposure to toxic substances during his service in Iraq.[222] But the more general point stands: in setting up the burn pits, administrators disregarded the effect that they would have upon not only the civilians but also the soldiers located nearby.

Contractually speaking, soldiers, by offering their services in exchange for a variety of benefits — from a stable salary, to healthcare, to education, to a pension — do in fact agree to follow orders. In the case of the mRNA shots, however, the loss of more than 8,000 persons from the active military was painted by lawmakers as harming national security, particularly in a time of flagging voluntary enlistments and failed recruitment campaigns, which have not managed to improve the image of the piggish "War on Terror," no matter how much lipstick is applied. The suicides of thousands of formerly healthy and happy troops have no doubt served as an effective anti-recruitment campaign for the past two decades, try though the public relations wing of the Pentagon may to burnish its image by pretending that the outcome of World War II absolves it from every U.S. government crime of mass homicide committed since 1945.

The military's COVID-19 vaccine mandate had already survived a variety of court challenges, thus demonstrating once again that scientific illiteracy is distributed throughout the populace at every socioeconomic stratum, including among persons in possession of a *Juris Doctor* (J.D.) degree. Nonetheless, thanks to the tireless efforts of Representative Massie, et al., the mandate was successfully outlawed by Congress as an appendage to the 3,854-page, gargantuan military budget in excess of $858 billion, which was signed into law by President Biden on December 23, 2022.[223] Press Secretary Karine Jean-Pierre expressed the expected lamentation to the effect that, by including the anti-mandate provision in the National Defense Authorization Act (NDAA), the Congress showed that it did not care about the health of the troops: "What we think happened here is that Republicans in Congress have decided that they'd rather fight against the health and well-being of our troops than protecting [*sic*] them."[224] Nonetheless, the mandate was indeed revoked, having been strategically appended to the piece of legislation most likely to pass each year, and which, for that reason, has become the place to tuck any and every provision which could never secure needed votes otherwise.

With the military mandate terminated by law, an ancillary debate rages on over whether the troops who refused to follow orders to roll up their sleeves should be compensated, or at least given back pay for the period during which they were essentially made into pariahs for asserting their right to bodily autonomy and refusing to serve as subjects in an experimental trial of a treatment of which they had no need. To date, the troops who lost their means of livelihood and suffered dismissal have not been compensated. This is because the government's own COVID-19 disinformation campaign plows ahead, undeterred by the data analyzed in a barrage of rapidly proliferating, peer-reviewed scientific studies.

Indeed, while the Pentagon has complied with the law to lift the mandate, it is nonetheless continuing to base deployments on vaccination status, again, as though the vaccines prevented both infection and transmission. In ending the mandate as required by law on January 10, 2023, Defense Secretary Lloyd Austin, too, claimed that the policy which he had imposed on August 24, 2021, had saved lives, and he issued a memo asserting the Pentagon's discretionary ability to continue to consider vaccination status in its daily operations:

> Other standing Departmental policies, procedures, and processes regarding immunizations remain in effect. These include the ability of commanders to consider, as appropriate, the individual immunization status of personnel in making deployment, assignment, and other operational decisions, including when vaccination is required for travel to, or entry into, a foreign nation.[225]

Both Defense Secretary Austin's and Press Secretary Jean-Pierre's insistence on perpetuating the government's 2021 narrative, according to which prior infection is somehow irrelevant to vaccination decisions, illustrated their failure to comprehend the intrinsic dependence of any effective vaccine on the tenability of the body's own immune system. That so many other people have failed to recognize the manifest absurdity of requiring people to undergo treatment for a disease which they have already survived is a testament to the scope and intensity of the marketing campaign of disinformation deployed against the populace over the past two years during the reign of public health guru Dr. Anthony Fauci.

Every vaccine in fact depends upon the human body's immune system in order to work. If the body's own immune system could not, in principle, fend off the invader, then no vaccine designed to prompt the immune system to fend off the invader could possibly work. Many of the persons who refused the shots, and were publicly denounced and denigrated by the government and media alike as "anti-vaxxers," did so on the entirely science-based grounds that their own bodies had already produced the antibodies and T-cells needed to fend off "severe illness and death," to borrow a turn of phrase from the White House Christmas 2021 message of impending doom directed toward unvaccinated persons.[226]

Before Congress acted to outlaw the military mandate, the OSHA (Occupational Safety and Health Administration) requirement imposed on companies with 100 employees or more had already been struck down on January 13, 2022, by the Supreme Court in a 6–3 ruling, ending the federal government's requirement of vaccination or weekly testing upon approximately 84 million persons.[227] In this case, too, however, the executive order was struck down neither because of concern with human rights and bodily autonomy, nor for the utter arbitrariness of such a requirement upon persons in firms with 100, but not 99, employees. Rather, the OSHA mandate was struck down as having overreached the stated purpose and intent of OSHA itself. The majority opinion reasoned that allowing the mandate to stand would bestow broad new powers upon the Office never granted to it by the legislature.

That justices on the Supreme Court which struck down the OSHA mandate were nonetheless under sway of the pro-vaccination propaganda, according to which the shots would stop the virus in its tracks, was clearly demonstrated by their decision to allow the HHS/CMS (Department of Health and Human Services, acting through the Centers for Medicare and Medicaid Services) mandate on healthcare workers to stand, in a 5–4 ruling, also on January 13, 2022.[228] Because healthcare workers had been exposed to the virus during the first year of the pandemic, many of them had already been infected with and recovered from COVID-19. The mandated vaccination of already recovered hospital and nursing home workers made no sense from the perspective of science, illustrating the very illogicality inherent to the military mandate. The nurses, orderlies, lab techs, and doctors who refused to comply with the mandate were in fact basing their decision on their professional training, according to which there is no better vaccine than the body's own recovery from infection by a virus, a position once championed by Anthony Fauci himself.[229]

One might reasonably presume that healthcare administrators should have at least a rudimentary understanding of immunology. And yet, defying any semblance of logic, somehow it came to be that vaccinated persons who were infected with COVID-19 were permitted to work, while unvaccinated persons who had already recovered from COVID-19 were forbidden from working in medical contexts. The fact that five out of nine Supreme Court justices saw fit to uphold the healthcare employee mandate was an indication not only that they sincerely wanted to protect patients, but also, more importantly, that they actually had no understanding of immunology.

It wasn't just Supreme Court justices who were hoodwinked by the redefinition of *vaccine* so as to imply that anyone who declined the mRNA shots was a selfish, ignorant *anti-vaxxer*. This harsh moral denunciation seemed justified in the minds of those who applied it, because they were operating under the assumption of the former definition, according to which any genuine vaccine would stop infection and transmission, and people who refused to undergo vaccination constituted, therefore, a public menace. The linguistic scenario represented an inverted case of Shakespeare's "A rose by any other name would smell as sweet." Millions of persons — from Supreme Court justices, to pundits in the mainstream media, to celebrities, to the press secretary and defense secretary themselves — were convinced that because the shots were called *vaccines*, this obviously implied that they stopped the spread of the virus.

In coming to terms with the stark statistical reality that the number of deaths from COVID-19 in fact *increased* after the widespread uptake of the "vaccines," we are left with two possibilities. We can continue to call the mRNA shots "vaccines" but qualify them as "very bad vaccines," or we can return to the earlier definition and acknowledge that they were never vaccines at all. "Vaccine" was just another pleasing label attached to a newly launched product in order to maximize its sales and to goad governments to impose mandates upon citizens against their will.

Viewed purely from a marketing perspective, the positive characterization of the experimental mRNA shots as "vaccines" was not unlike the inclusion of package inserts in boxes of Oxycontin asserting that the new class of narcotic painkiller was nonaddictive and, moreover, resistant to abuse. By now, it has become undeniable that the unscrupulous marketing ploys used by pharmaceutical companies to maximize sales of narcotics, which were fully condoned by the FDA (Food and Drug Administration), fueled the opioid addiction crisis in the years after the launch of Oxycontin, leading ultimately to an epidemic of narcotics overdose deaths.

Now that the populace has confused "shots" with "vaccines" for more than two years — and indeed people regularly refer to the flu shot as a "vaccine," despite its middling efficacy — it would seem that the honorific term will continue to be applied to any elixir which is being promoted by the powerful pharma-government alliance. This use of neologism or rebranding does not bode well for the future of free persons, given the explicitly stated plans in the works to require "vaccine passports" for international travel. By loosening the definition of "vaccine" to include whatever the powers that be wish for their subjects to ingest, we are careening toward a dystopian *Brave New World* in which citizens are required by law to dose themselves with substances or suffer dire consequences if they resist. The threat of job loss and cutting off access to their very own bank accounts were two of the sticks already brandished by governments during the Coronapocalypse, in addition to the refusal to allow non-compliant persons to cross borders.

As though in the throes of yet another senior moment, President Biden, who had declared the pandemic "over" back in September 2022, announced in mid-December 2022 that every U.S. household would be eligible once again (as he had announced at about the same time the previous year) for "free" COVID-19 tests to be delivered to their doorstep for at-home use.[230] Predictably enough, after Biden's magnanimous provision of "free" test kits (funded by taxpayers) to every household, on December 30, 2022, the TSA (Transportation Security Administration) quietly extended its Emergency Order requiring vaccination of any person attempting to ford U.S. shores.[231] The new order is set to expire on April 10, 2023, with the same rare exceptions admitted, including for those who wish to immigrate to the United States. Anyone attempting to visit relatives not seen now for years, or to do some tourism, must first demonstrate that he or she has been "fully vaccinated." Let us briefly review the actual "public health" implications of this requirement.

According to the TSA order, vaccinated travelers infected with COVID-19 may enter the United States — this follows from the fact that there is no testing requirement on anyone in possession of proof of having been fully vaccinated. Many vaccinated persons (including President and First Lady Biden) have become infected with COVID-19. Therefore, any vaccinated person, including those attempting to enter the United States, may in fact be infected with the virus. QED.

Unvaccinated travelers who do not carry the virus, however, as could be demonstrated through a negative test, may not enter the United States, nor may persons previously infected who have fully recovered from a bout of the wild virus and therefore definitively demonstrated their ability to survive infection. Note that a number of other countries (Brazil, China, Colombia, Nicaragua, et al.) continue to require *either* proof of vaccination *or* a negative test, a policy which at least has the semblance of common sense and consistency, under the assumption that the shots do in fact prevent infection and transmission — which we now know that they do not. But the point is that, if the shots prevented infection and transmission, then it would at least not be completely illogical to require testing of the unvaccinated. Three countries remain closed to all visitors, whether vaccinated or unvaccinated: Libya, Turkmenistan, and Yemen. Ten countries currently require unvaccinated persons both to test and to quarantine in order to enter. (The entry requirements have changed frequently since 2020 but are regularly updated on the Kayak countries map.[232])

In contrast, the U.S. requirement defies all logic, at least from the perspective of public health, showing that we have truly entered into *Nineteen Eighty-Four* territory, with government officials regularly spouting out nonsensical locutions such as 2 + 2 = 5 and expecting the citizenry to applaud in response and parrot the pronouncements throughout social media. Preposterously, a non-citizen who underwent vaccination two years ago may enter the United States, while someone who recovered from the virus six months ago may not enter. Yet anyone who dares to point out that the government's policies contradict the deliverances of empirical science continues to be shamed by the president, the press secretary, and many in the media and the populace who have been taken in by what is manifestly a ruse.

The requirement of COVID-19 vaccination on persons entering the United States serves, in reality, only two purposes: first, to punish those who refused to comply with the ubiquitous propaganda campaign to inoculate everyone everywhere with an experimental mRNA elixir; and, second, and most ominously, to normalize the notion that governments have and should have the authority to tell people which medications they must ingest. There is no sense in which the TSA requirement and the associated ongoing State of Emergency are supported by either theories of science or the statistical evidence amassed since 2020. Instead, "vaccination" has become a badge of compliance, which those indoctrinated continue to believe should be required of all others, against their will.

It's not over 'til it's over.

24. This Was a Test of the Emergency Use Authorization System

February 27, 2023
Holladay, Utah

Data continues to emerge according to which, not only were the mRNA shots ineffective at preventing infection and transmission of COVID-19, but they may have caused widespread harm to persons cajoled or coerced into undergoing vaccination, despite their own relative invulnerability to the worst effects of the virus.[233] Anecdotal cases abound, but diehard regime narrative devotees continue to dismiss such "incidents" — thousands of which are recorded in the government's own VAERS (Vaccine Adverse Effects Reporting System) database — as purely coincidental. It is more difficult to downplay reports involving entire cohorts, such as the increased incidence of myocarditis among young males, which the CDC itself has acknowledged.[234] Some critics have suggested that a disproportionately high percentage of pregnant women in Pfizer's initial trial of the shots suffered miscarriages.

Back in November 2021, in the midst of the widespread, aggressive "Vaccinate everyone!" campaign, I spoke with a woman in Oregon who matter-of-factly mentioned that her (vaccinated) daughter had suffered three recent miscarriages. Recognizing that it was too late to do anything anyway, given that the daughter had already been vaccinated, I did not dare to suggest that her troubles may have been caused by the shots she had no doubt been exhorted by her doctor to take. At that time, following the lead of CDC director Rochelle Walensky, health officials everywhere were in the midst of a marketing blitz according to which COVID-19 vaccination would protect mothers and their babies alike.

I said nothing to the woman in Oregon about the dangers of introducing foreign substances into pregnant women (although I had written about it — see Chapter 8), but I did naturally wonder at the time whether there might be a causal connection between the poor daughter's miscarriages and the shots, given the biological activity of the spike protein already known to induce blood clotting and heart troubles. The mother of the young woman — who was pregnant again, for a fourth time — seemed optimistic that somehow there was nothing to worry about, even after three failed attempts to bring a baby into the world. It is possible, I realized then and continue to own, as I must, that the woman was simply unable, for unrelated reasons, to carry a child to term. But given that the biologically active spike protein is what the original virus used to access cells, and production of lots of it was induced by the injected mRNA, it would not take a tinfoil hat conspiracy theorist to surmise that the pregnancies may have been sabotaged by the shots.

Critics such as feminist scholar Naomi Wolf, who early on in the pandemic raised questions about the shot's safety, given the many reports of irregular menstrual cycles in women who underwent vaccination,[235] were denounced as purveyors of misinformation and immediately deplatformed by the social media giants. Only recently have such "conspiracy theorists" been permitted to articulate their concerns in the public sphere once again — and only on some platforms, including Twitter, which to Elon Musk's credit reinstated thousands of accounts shut down for the crime of deviating from the narrative favored by the pharma-government alliance. If the shots are indeed dangerous to fetuses, it is, needless to say, too late for all of the pregnant women tricked into believing that because the CDC insisted that there was no evidence of risk to them and their offspring, they should therefore roll up their sleeves.

That Pfizer knew all along that their mRNA shots had effects upon women's hormonal systems was corroborated through a Project Veritas sting operation involving a Pfizer research director, Jordon Trishton Walker.[236] In the recorded interview thought by him to be a friendly conversation with a date, Walker observed that the shots seemed somehow to be affecting the endocrine systems of women. The delicate hormonal balance needed to maintain a pregnancy suggests an immediate connection between the widely reported menstruation irregularities of women and the incidence of miscarriages in some of the initial trial subjects.

The data interpreted by some critics to imply that miscarriage was one of the many possible side effects of the Pfizer shot were made public only recently, with the release of a large trove of court-ordered documents which the company is now required by law to provide, despite its initial insistence that it would take seventy-five years to do so. Setting aside the question of whether miscarriage is in fact a side effect of the shots, the very idea that it would take so many years to make public the documents said to have served as the basis for the FDA's (Food and Drug Administration's) decision to grant the Pfizer product Emergency Use Authorization (EUA) so that it could forego the customarily stringent multi-year testing program required of pharmaceutical products more generally, struck many people as absurd.

To my mind, the situation constituted a classic Charybdis and Scylla. If it was humanly impossible to process and assess all of the data (all 400,000 pages of it) in the short period between the creation of the vaccines and December 11, 2020, when the EUA was granted, this could be taken to imply that the persons on the committee incompetently executed their role and indeed based their decision to approve the shots primarily on Pfizer's obvious wish that they do so. Alternatively, it was always possible to process the documents for publication, and the company's resistance to doing so was due to the contents of the documents themselves, which might harm the ambitious sales program to vaccinate everyone on the planet with the new product.

The director of the CDC, Rochelle Walensky, encouraged pregnant women from the beginning to get the shots, quite deceptively claiming that there was no cause for worry about possible health risks to fetuses. The safety information provided with the original shots itself indicated that pregnant women had been excluded from the initial trials, as they are for most pharmaceutical products. The reason why pregnant women are not included in early-stage clinical trials of products intended for the general population is that they represent a special case, given the fragile chemical environment enveloping the fetus. It is a matter of common knowledge that developing human beings are highly sensitive to, and often endangered by, foreign substances — alcohol and nicotine being two well-documented examples. The vulnerability of fetuses was most notoriously and unforgettably demonstrated when pregnant women were prescribed Thalidomide on the basis of clinical trials which, again, excluded pregnant women. As in the case of the COVID-19 vaccines, Thalidomide was distributed by doctors under the misleading marketing line that there was no evidence that it would harm fetuses. Thalidomide killed thousands of babies and deformed thousands more before it was finally withdrawn from the market.

We now know from recently released Pfizer safety data that some of the women in the initial trial were in fact pregnant — apparently without having known that this was the case at the time, which was why they were not excluded from the trial. The vaccines may or may not have caused their reported miscarriages, but the fact that the CDC would encourage pregnant women, on the basis of nearly no data, to undergo vaccination betrays a reckless disregard and their true goals in injecting everyone everywhere, even members of low-risk cohorts, with the mRNA treatment. Ignorance is bliss for pharmaceutical companies, which can continue to market and sell products for years, reaping billions of dollars of profits, before finally halting sales on the basis of widely reported and what come eventually to be undeniable post-launch problems, as in the cases of Vioxx,[237] Belviq,[238] Baycol,[239] etc.

Above and beyond the profit motive was plausibly the desire to test the newfangled mRNA technology on the largest sample of human beings possible — whether or not those injected actually needed any treatment whatsoever in contending with COVID-19. Of course, if the desire on the part of Pfizer CEO Albert Bourla and Moderna CEO Stéphane Bancel was to make strides ahead in the research and development of other lucrative medications, then the quest for data, too, was ultimately driven by the profit motive — albeit looking forward, to future possible blockbuster drugs.

Certainly, the steadfast resistance — indeed, the outright refusal — on the part of public health authorities such as Dr. Anthony Fauci and Dr. Rochelle Walensky, for more than a year after the launch of the COVID-19 vaccines, to acknowledge the relevance of natural immunity in those persons previously infected, and to recommend appropriate adjustments to the U.S. government's mandates for both healthcare workers and military personnel, supports the hypothesis that one of the overarching aims of the aggressive, relentless vaccine campaign was not to save the lives of the small percentage of human beings vulnerable to the virus, but rather to amass data.

Corroborating this interpretation, according to which the companies hoped not only to reap a windfall of profits but also to collect a huge amount of data, is the explanation by many critics (including Robert F. Kennedy, Jr., and Dr. Peter McCullough) of the assiduous suppression of any and every alternative therapeutic which the vaccine salespersons recognized would compete with and diminish the uptake of the newly patented products. Most importantly of all, ivermectin and hydroxychloroquine were dismissed and denounced by public health authorities, and ridiculed by parroting pundits throughout the media, because EUA cannot be granted to products when alternative therapies are available.

In his conversation with a Project Veritas reporter, Dr. Jordon Trishton Walker also shared the potentially explosive piece of information that Pfizer executives had floated ideas such as mutating the COVID-19 virus so as to be able to develop vaccines preemptively. It was not entirely clear from Walker's remarks whether the intention would be to release those mutated viruses to direct the course of the disease in populations, or simply to predict which variants would pop up on the scene naturally through mutations of the virus in its effort to self-propagate by evading the antibodies induced by the latest shots.

Pfizer responded to the bombshell revelation by effectively minimizing the story through suggesting that the process described by their (now former, I presume) employee was essentially part of the normal, necessary research conducted in producing, for example, the flu shot each year. Nearly everyone by now is more or less aware that the flu shot is a gamble, involving researchers predicting which strains will be most prevalent and virulent. People who undergo inoculation against those versions may still fall ill because they may or may not come in contact with the predicted dominant strains. Some individuals report anecdotally that they were never more ill than during a year when they opted for the "free" flu shot, which clearly indicates that they encountered versions of the pathogen not expected by the researchers who determined the ingredients for the products distributed during that particular flu season. Unsurprisingly, neither anecdotal reports, nor adverse effects, nor even consistently poor efficacy rates have deterred pharmaceutical firms from pushing for widespread uptake of their mediocre flu shot products in very public and misleading advertising campaigns fronted by government health authorities.

If Pfizer's intention in mutating the COVID-19 virus was to release it into the human population in order to induce countless numbers of persons to seek protection by purchasing (or obtaining from their government) the "vaccine" developed in order to stop that strain, then that would constitute a flagrant violation of any decent person's basic sense of ethics. Such a possibility would moreover, and disconcertingly, be taken by some to accrue a degree of plausibility to the conspiratorial notion according to which the original COVID-19 virus was not only a gain-of-function product, created by researchers in a lab, but also intentionally released into the world in order to initiate the "Great Reset" being promoted by members of the World Economic Forum (WEF), led by Klaus Schwab.

More plausible, I believe, is that Pfizer and Moderna, et al., are primarily focused on the future of their other new mRNA products in the works. It is not at all far-fetched to surmise that the relentless, divisive push to vaccinate everyone everywhere with the first mRNA treatment ever tested on a population of human beings, made possible *only* by the FDA's EUA, was spearheaded by companies with much broader goals in mind. The CEOs of these companies have publicly vaunted their plans to use mRNA to cure cancer and other intractable diseases, which in fact best explains their manifest fervor to acquire as much data as possible, by all means necessary. Such a program, albeit less explicitly heinous than creating illnesses in order to be able to sell patented cures for the symptoms caused by them, nonetheless involved using all of the people coerced into undergoing treatments of which they had no need as the means to the companies' mercenary ends.

Further evidence for this admittedly unsavory interpretation can be seen in the push to vaccinate children, even infants, despite the minimal danger posed to them by the COVID-19 virus. If, in reality, the chance of a child dying from COVID-19 is less than the chance of being hit by a bolt of lightning, then it is hard to see why anyone would push for uptake under a public health pretext. Yet those who wish to foist the product on young persons, including infants, have continued to press the line according to which the virus poses a serious health risk to everyone, and the vaccine will help to protect children, along with their parents. This despite data according to which the protection provided by the shots, even to the vulnerable persons who might be said to benefit, plummets to nothing after only a few months. (Preposterously enough, according to one recent study at the Cleveland Clinic, in the long term, the more shots one has received, the greater one's chances of contracting COVID-19![240])

A second reason why children have been important for the product companies is peculiar to the United States, where the PREP (Public Readiness and Emergency Preparedness) Act protecting companies from liability in the event of adverse effects covers any product approved as a part of the child immunization schedule. Demonstrating their complete capture by pharmaceutical industry forces, on February 9, 2023, the CDC added the COVID-19 shots to the long list of those recommended in the childhood vaccination schedule (which now includes dozens of shots[241]), thus ensuring the product companies massive profits for years to come through the inoculation of persons not at significant risk from the virus, using a product whose already nearly negligible protective capacity for invulnerable persons (a risk reduction of ~1% — or less[242]) spans less than a few months.

Unbelievably enough, the new CDC recommendation for children (beginning at six months) includes the original COVID-19 vaccine (though the wild strain of the virus may no longer exist), along with booster shots, for which the only clinical trial on human beings is currently underway — on the millions of persons who rolled up their sleeves on the basis of safety data gathered from only animal trials. The results are trickling in on the first round of "bivalent" booster shots, which have so far been demonstrated to have middling (30%) efficacy in preventing infection by the variant they are intended to address.[243] But the virus will continue to mutate, thus serving as the pretext for producing new booster formulas. This implies that, under the CDC's immunization guidelines, each new booster shot will of necessity constitute yet another experimental trial, to be conducted, shockingly enough, upon children throughout the years of their development into adults. In other words, children have been set up to serve as test subjects (i.e., human guinea pigs) for each newly developed "booster" to follow in the future as the virus continues to mutate, despite the fact that children constitute the least vulnerable cohort of them all.

Why should "vaccines" which do not offer long-term immunity to anyone and are not even necessary for children — the CDC itself explicitly claims that most children will experience only mild symptoms from COVID-19 — be included in the battery of time-tested vaccines such as those against polio, measles, etc.? Along with the desire to sell products and to be able to test new products on children is, again, scandalously enough, the fact that the CDC's addition of the mRNA shots to the children's immunization schedule protects the manufacturers in perpetuity from lawsuits, even after the State of Emergency has ended. President Biden has announced that the State of Emergency will be lifted on May 11, 2023, two months *after* the CDC added the COVID-19 shots to the children's immunization schedule.

Because state and local officials follow the cues of the CDC, we can expect to see its recommendation for childhood inoculation by the COVID-19 shots swiftly transformed into mandates for public school children in states throughout the country. This will likely happen in places such as Massachusetts, California, and New York, where health authorities have persisted in retaining laws which restrict the behavior of residents even as new data continues to refute the erroneous premises widely embraced by officials in the spring of 2020 regarding masks, social distancing, etc. States such as Florida rescinded the COVID-19 emergency laws, and have passed legislation to protect children, but the fact remains: with the federal level CDC recommendation in place, the product companies will retain their protection from future litigation arising from adverse effects, even if the data currently being collected and analyzed eventually demonstrate widespread harm to either children or adults.

It would be a mistake to judge corporations by the moral standards appropriate to individual persons. Corporations are beholden only to their stockholders, and their sole goal is to maximize profit. But the spokespersons for such companies are themselves individual human beings, as are all of the authorities representing public health organizations whose ostensible *raison d'être* is to protect members of society, not to maximize the profits of their sponsors. When institutions such as the FDA are coopted by mercenary forces, they cease to perform the function which citizens are depending upon them to execute. Because this already happened in the case of the opioid crisis, the fact that people fell for the trick once again in the case of the COVID-19 "vaccines" is best and perhaps only explained by the fearmongering campaign used to traumatize them psychologically to the point where they lost all critical bearings and agreed to undergo an experimental treatment of which most of them had no need.

25. Launched on a Wing and a Prayer, for Billions of Dollars

March 14, 2023
Holladay, Utah

Way back in the spring of 2020, the provocative title of an article caught my eye. Upon reading it, I learned that researchers were rushing to create a vaccine before the COVID-19 virus mutated, which would render the vaccine nugatory and destroy all hopes of creating a blockbuster panacea. Curious at the time, such a warning can be viewed today as having been prophetic. (Note: That article, which offered a business slant on the historic vaccine competition, is no longer available through Google — "*some results have been removed*," and are seemingly irretrievable — but here's one with a similar title from April 2020: "Coronavirus mutation could threaten the race to develop vaccine."[244])

Consider the stunning conclusion of a peer-reviewed scientific journal article published in January 2023:

> Viruses that replicate in the human respiratory mucosa without infecting systemically, including influenza A, SARS-CoV-2, endemic coronaviruses, RSV, and many other "common cold" viruses, cause significant mortality and morbidity and are important public health concerns. Because these viruses generally do not elicit complete and durable protective immunity by themselves, they have not to date been effectively controlled by licensed or experimental vaccines.[245]

Accustomed as everyone is by now to a relentless barrage of contradictory proclamations and retaliatory responses to them, the claim that mRNA was never fit for purpose against rapidly mutating coronaviruses might be written off by the usual suspects as the ravings of yet another anti-vaxxer conspiracy theorist. Except that this paper was co-authored by Dr. Anthony Fauci, the most visible and persistent pusher of the newfangled COVID-19 vaccines throughout 2021 and 2022. So what happened?

Against all conventional wisdom on the ethical practice of medicine,[246] Fauci did everything in his power to achieve maximal uptake of an experimental treatment by human beings across all cohorts, without regard to patient health, age, or any other identifying factor beyond their possession of an arm into which to inject a novel product granted Emergency Use Authorization (EUA) after an accelerated review by the Food and Drug

Administration (FDA). Not only did Fauci ignore the vast disparities in vulnerability to severe illness and death between healthy infants and frail nonagenarians, but he also conducted himself for two years as though natural immunity through previous infection were somehow irrelevant to the question of whether a patient should roll up his sleeve.

Now, in the light of Fauci's own published scientific findings, it would appear that he was right, in a sense, about natural immunity all along, albeit in an unexpectedly perverse way. First of all, as we already witnessed in real time, coronaviruses as a class, including SARS-CoV-2 (COVID-19), mutate rapidly in order to propagate themselves. This "discovery" served as the basis for the development of "boosters," which, it was claimed, became necessary when "fully vaccinated" persons continued to become infected with COVID-19. Major outbreak-inducing strains such as Delta and Omicron, which arise through mutation, will always be one step ahead of last year's vaccines, having survived precisely by evading the antibodies induced by injections of the previous virus generation's mRNA.

According to Fauci's own findings, however, there is a second, even more compelling reason for denying that either vaccine or natural immunity to COVID-19 can ever be permanent. The primary difference between diseases such as measles, for which vaccines work, and the seasonal flu or SARS-CoV-2, for which they do not, is that the body's natural immune response rises only to the level of the severity of the pathogen. Since most people can survive coronaviruses, the minimal response needed to defeat the invader is rather mild, which is why immunity dissipates rapidly over time and people can become reinfected again and again, even if they have recovered from natural infection, and whether or not they have undergone vaccination.

There are, of course, people who die of the flu or COVID-19, but they nearly always have comorbidities or weaknesses which make them vulnerable to a pathogen that healthy bodies are capable of defeating. Notwithstanding the massive propaganda campaign for universal vaccination, most healthy young persons would have survived COVID-19, and would not have been hospitalized, with or without vaccination. Given the abundance of statistical evidence, there is simply no sense in which it can be truthfully asserted that healthy young persons with no comorbidities were "saved" by the shots. On the other hand, extremely frail and elderly persons can indeed be killed by the virus, regardless of how many "vaccines" they have taken. When it comes to the mercurial class of coronaviruses — instantiated by not only the common cold and the seasonal flu, but also COVID-19 — so-called vaccines will never transcend their pedestrian identity as mere shots, for they are constitutionally incapable of offering long-term protection, not only because these viruses rapidly mutate, but also, and more fundamentally, because the body's natural response to infection by such transitory viruses is never robust enough to be permanent. Just as having survived the flu one year has nearly no bearing on whether one will contract another case of the flu, from a different variant, in the future, no so-called vaccine solution to COVID-19 can confer long-lasting protection.

Take as many boosters as you like, until the end of time, but having done so may or may not prevent you from contracting the latest iteration of the virus — or protect anyone else — since every booster or flu shot is the result of researchers' "best guess" of what the specific properties of the next generation of viruses will be. It appears, then, that the widely celebrated and aggressively marketed, and in some cases mandated, COVID-19 "vaccines," fully funded by the tax-paying recipients of "free" shots, were in fact launched on a wing and a prayer. There was really no hope all along that the shots would or could offer long-term protection, although it was claimed for marketing purposes that they were highly effective and would save millions of lives. That those selling points were in fact lies may explain why they were supplemented all along the way with such eerily self-contradictory slogans as: "The vaccinated need to be protected from the unvaccinated!"

Dr. Fauci's surprising publication reveals that the abundant optimism exuded by him and others in attempting to maximize vaccine uptake was scientifically unfounded from the beginning. Neither the mRNA technology nor the traditional vaccines (which introduce a small amount of the live or dead pathogen into the body to elicit an immune response) can be effective in the case of rapidly evolving pathogens such as coronaviruses, against which the highly efficient human body mounts the minimal needed response. But this is hardly news, for we already knew long before 2020 that, despite assiduous efforts spanning decades, no one ever managed to develop a vaccine against the common cold. Likewise, the widely touted flu shots, marketed in very public ad campaigns only slightly less aggressive than those for the COVID-19 treatments, are in fact mediocre at best, as Fauci himself has averred.

If vaccine technology, whether vector- or mRNA-based, is simply a mismatch for the nature of rapidly mutating viruses, and this is a matter of common knowledge, readily accessible to anyone working in virology, then how are we to understand Fauci's comportment throughout the Coronapocalypse? And why did he and his coauthors boldly reaffirm in January 2023 what many other researchers have been saying for years, including a few brave souls who were silenced when they tried to suggest the same from 2020 to 2022?

Fauci faces something of a "Charybdis or Scylla?" dilemma here, for if he was ignorant of basic truths of immunology known by competent and knowledgeable scientists before 2020, then he had no business serving as the nation's fount of public health wisdom. Double-masked Fauci devotees, in the aftermath of what was empirically indistinguishable from a full-scale psyop spanning more than two years, will no doubt remain reluctant to renounce their allegiance to the person who, they believe, "guided" us through the pandemic. Confronted with the revelations of Fauci et al.'s January 2023 publication, such followers may most charitably conclude that the object of their reverence did genuinely believe in the mRNA vaccines and continues to follow "The Science" where it leads, in this case, to acknowledge failure.

That Fauci honestly did not know that the mRNA shots would never work has also been the conclusion of a few of his most vociferous critics, including Alex Berenson, who somewhat ironically was spurned as "The Pandemic's Wrongest Man" by *The Atlantic* back in April 2021.[247] (Morally speaking, that title surely belongs to Dr. Anthony Fauci himself, for the sheer brazenness with which he defied all known principles of medical ethics in pushing for universal vaccination across all cohorts.) Berenson was banned from social media under pressure by no less a power than the U.S. government itself, when he dared to question the Fauci script at the height of the Coronapocalyptic hysteria. (Berenson's lawsuit alleging the government's violation of his First Amendment right to free speech is pending.[248])

Notwithstanding the superficial appeal (and attendant *Schadenfreude*) of the "Fauci was ignorant and is now eating crow" hypothesis, the Scylla horn of the interpretive dilemma would seem to cohere far better with the character of a man who remarkably responded to his critics on national television that "You're really attacking not only Dr. Anthony Fauci; you're attacking science."[249] Such a person is not someone whom we would ordinarily regard as endowed with the humility needed to admit either ignorance or error. To my mind (and others, such as Dr. Robert Malone, agree[250]), Fauci's recent publication is yet another gambit perfectly consistent with his comportment throughout the pandemic. While Fauci's admission that the mRNA technology is not fit for purpose against coronaviruses may on its face seem surprising, in fact, it is entirely true to form.

Yes, Fauci's gambit is most plausibly interpreted as the latest chapter in his time-tested "fail forward" playbook: to use the outcome of the COVID-19 shot experiment to rally for yet more funding for the pharmaceutical industry. Like all good bureaucrats, Fauci uses government fiascos as a springboard to increase the reach and budget of his domain. In other words, Fauci, having quite effectively painted the COVID-19 virus as the most evil bogeyman of them all, is simply continuing his efforts to impel politicians to dole out *even more* billions of dollars to the government-boosted industry which he has loyally supported throughout his entire career, as has been ably documented by Robert F. Kennedy, Jr.[251] In addition to being consistent with Fauci's dismissive, smug, and seemingly shameless character, this interpretation coheres well with the general *modus operandi* of the pharmaceutical industry, which has displayed in recent decades an uncanny capacity to "fail forward" by pivoting and innovating so as to reap massive profits even when their products generate consequences worse than the conditions which they were intended to address.

Note that slippery snake oil salesmen such as Pfizer's CEO Albert Bourla carefully calibrated their pitches from the beginning in order to protect themselves from future allegations of fraud by equivocating about the "efficacy" of their COVID-19 treatments. When directly questioned in December 2020 about the vaccine's ability to limit transmission of the virus, Bourla offered casual, off-the-cuff replies such as, "I think that's something that needs to be examined. We're not certain about that right now."[252] His colleague, Uğur Şahin (co-founder and CEO of BioNTech), cagily couched his anticipatory optimism in these terms: "The first interim analysis of our global Phase 3 study provides evidence that a vaccine *may* effectively prevent COVID-19"[253] [my emphasis]. The rest is history. When it later emerged, to the surprise of everyone whose understanding of the crisis was shaped exclusively by the Pfizer-sponsored mainstream media, that the company never even tested the shots for their ability to prevent transmission, gaslighting fact-checkers rushed to the defense of the executives.[254] *Why in the world would anyone ever have believed that the new vaccines would prevent transmission and infection?*

The government-subsidized pharma giants succeeded in profiting enormously from the politically amplified crisis by persistently touting the efficacy of their products against a virus which 99+% of people were perfectly capable of surviving on their own. The shot salesmen claimed victory when injected persons did not die, when in reality most of them would have survived even if they had declined the treatment or been injected with an inert placebo instead. But the scheme ultimately worked, because marketers (including public health authorities such as Anthony Fauci and Rochelle Walensky) unerringly referred to the shots as "vaccines," a piece of sleight of hand made possible by the CDC's own diluted redefinition of the term in 2021 to mean "a preparation that is *used to stimulate the body's immune response against diseases*."[255] This linguistic legerdemain worked wonders to promote the new shots, when in fact the new definition is so broad and open-ended as to make it possible to label as a *vaccine* anything that strengthens the immune system, including leafy green vegetables, vitamins C and D, etc.

In retrospect, there can be no doubt that the populace and the politicians crafting policy all assumed that the labeling of the mRNA treatment as *vaccines* implied that the shots stopped transmission and infection, even while the savviest of the snake oil salesmen evinced ignorance from the start about the most important question of all: whether these "vaccines" were indeed like all of the other vaccines, capable not just of "stimulating" the immune system, but of producing dependable and durable immunity.

Given the statistics now available, even the more modest claim, continually chanted by pharma marketers and their lackeys in the media, that the mRNA treatment greatly diminished severe illness and hospitalization, may have been false. For the death toll of COVID-19 victims increased rather than decreased in the year after the "vaccine" launch, and the countries with the worst vaccine uptake had some of the best outcomes. On top of the virus deaths, thousands of people were diagnosed with post-vaccine injuries of a variety of sorts, believed by many of them, their families, and at least some of their doctors to have been caused by the shots. Some of the vaccine-injured ended up dying long before their time, and excess deaths were also caused by the disastrous political response to the virus, with fatal drug overdoses reaching record levels. Millions of persons missed vital health screenings, having been terrorized into believing that they could not leave their homes (much less enter COVID-19-infested health facilities!) without contracting something akin to the Black Plague. Among those who sought help for their ailments, some were flat-out denied treatment for acute illnesses, either because they were not dying specifically of COVID-19, or because they had refused the experimental treatment.

In coming to terms with what transpired over the past three years, it is helpful to bear in mind pre-2020 history. When the pharmaceutical industry's newfangled psychotropic medications did not work as advertised, they created and blitz-marketed "add-on" drugs to increase the efficacy of antidepressants now known to have exhibited success in clinical trials on a par with placebos, but with far worse long-term adverse effects, up to and including addiction and suicidal ideation. Similarly, the slick pivot of the industry in response to the opioid catastrophe (caused by the industry itself[256]) was to launch and market drugs which could help people in the throes of narcotics addiction.

The flu shots marketed in collaboration with and subsidized by governments have been demonstrated in clinical trials to succeed on a par with placebos, while post-flu shot deaths are invariably written off as "coincidental." Nonetheless, the industry capitalizes on the fact that they are starting anew each year — the previous year's flu shot results being irrelevant to the next year's projected success. As a result, when heavily lobbied and propagandized authorities impose mandates in some places (such as the State of Massachusetts), this may lead others to follow suit. Crony capitalist windfall profits ensure the ever-augmenting marketing budget of pharma firms, with the result that each subsequent year's sales will exceed the previous year's tally.

Given such precedents, no one should be surprised if the failure of the COVID-19 shots to prevent infection and transmission, or even to diminish the number of persons who died from the virus, does indeed end up serving as the pretext for governments to infuse even more money into research and development of new and what are promised once again to be "miraculous" cures to be used in the future. Not long after the launch of the COVID-19 vaccines, auxiliary treatments such as Pfizer's Paxlovid and Merck's Lagevrio were developed to treat people who became infected with the virus despite having been "fully" vaccinated. As clear evidence that many people's capacity for critical thought continues to be compromised by fear, when legislation to rescind the utterly illogical and unscientific COVID-19 vaccine mandate on foreigners entering the United States made it to the floor of the House of Representatives, 201 Democratic congresspersons voted to keep the executive order in place.

The ongoing support of the official government pro-pharma narrative by the president, the press secretary, the defense secretary, and most Democratic members of Congress, even in the face of ample evidence (including post-vaccination positive COVID-19 tests) demonstrating that the shots did not diminish the incidence of infection, is best explained by the fact that policymakers prefer not to own up to their mistakes. Ordinarily, individuals base their future actions on what they have learned from past experience. The question arises in the present circumstance: *Why is there still a push for vaccine passports when the COVID-19 vaccines do not in fact confer immunity?* The assumptions funding the push for universal vaccination continue to be embraced, as though the vaccines worked resplendently, despite an accumulation of scientific evidence to the contrary.

Now that Fauci himself has clearly explained why the mRNA technology will never offer a lasting solution to COVID-19, why would anyone, including Joe Biden and other advocates for the WHO (World Health Organization), still be in favor of implementing a universal health passport system regulating the movement of persons throughout the world? The current crop of shots does not offer long-term protection and does not moderate illness, except in the case of persons in a very narrow cohort. Why require any persons to demonstrate that they participated in the experimental mRNA trial more than two years ago in order to be able to enter a country where the circulating variants bear little resemblance to the strain used to determine the formula of the first crop of vaccines?

There is no plausible health pretext available to explain why political leaders around the world would be keen to impose such a restrictive health passport program on free people, preventing them from traveling unless they first demonstrate their willingness to comply with future possible arbitrary orders decreed by public health authorities. That anyone not holding pharma stocks would support at this point the adoption of a health passport is best explained, again, by the politically induced trauma which appears to have psychologically scarred some persons for life. But just as the failure of the lockdowns to "Stop the spread!" impelled leaders at every level of government — local, state, and federal — to prolong and intensify the lockdowns, those who pushed vaccine mandates will continue to press for universal vaccination passport requirements under the flatly false assumption that the reason why so many people died of COVID-19 was the evil anti-vaxxers' refusal to comply.

What we are witnessing, the in some ways strangely intransigent push for vaccine passports, is entirely consistent with the comportment of the very persons who just succeeded in selling billions of shots. They will continue to insist that what we need to do is provide even more government funding to the pharmaceutical industry so that they can develop more and better cures for our ills. As disturbing as this may be, the most plausible explanation for the vigorous attempt to impose a health credential system on the people of the world is to provide the pharmaceutical industry with a limitless supply of not only customers, but also future experimental subjects.

As we have seen (in Chapter 24), the addition of the COVID-19 shot to the CDC's immunization schedule for children — whose chances of dying from the virus are minuscule — serves only industry interests, by ensuring an endless crop of healthy young arms into which to inject the latest and greatest snake oils claimed to be panaceas (until it emerges that they are not). Likewise, the implementation of a universal health passport scheme restricting the motion of persons who opt not to undergo medical treatments of which they have no need would not only reap massive profits to the pharmaceutical industry, but also represent the dawning of the pharma-techno state, in which citizens are subjects whose bodies are owned by their governments.

26. The Crony Capitalist Origins of Our Oligarchy

March 28, 2023
Holladay, Utah

Republicans have of late been setting the stage for war with China, which would seem to explain the sudden interest — after years of apathy on the part of nearly everyone but Senator Rand Paul — in determining the origins of the COVID-19 virus. Was or was not the deadly bug which upended the entire world released from the Wuhan Institute of Virology? Was or was not the creation of SARS-CoV-2 funded by the U.S. government, and made possible by gain-of-function research advocate Dr. Anthony Fauci, the very person appointed to lead the country's pandemic response? Or perhaps the origin of the virus was entirely natural — a pangolin kissed a turtle, or something along those lines — and the rest is history.

Early inquiries about the matter were ridiculed, shut down, and even denounced as "racist" back when Trump was president. *How dare Trump call COVID-19 "The China virus"?!*[257] The Biden administration, however, has made "anti-China" sentiment acceptable again, which explains why both the U.S. Senate and the U.S. House of Representatives voted in a rare show of unanimity to declassify all intelligence relating to the question of virus origins. Why such documents were ever classified in the first place should emerge in due course, assuming that the Biden administration actually abides by the law. President Biden signed the legislation on March 20, 2023, but offered the following qualification:

> In implementing this legislation, my Administration will declassify and share as much of that information as possible, consistent with my constitutional authority to protect against the disclosure of information that would harm national security.[258]

What the recent unanimous vote by Congress reveals is that, while there may be superficial differences between the reds and the blues, those differences are akin to rounding errors, given the War Party duopoly's unerring support of the military, including the budget ratified each year in the National Defense Authorization Act (NDAA), which is on track to exceed $1 trillion in the not-too-distant future. Both the Senate and the House of Representatives lavish funds upon the Department of Defense and prioritize the support of war above anything and everything else. Given the difference in magnitude between military and non-military outlays, most discretionary spending debates between Republicans and Democrats have become petty squabbles over chump change.

The spigot of money and weapons for the Ukraine-Russia conflict has yet to be turned off, but a warmaker's job is never done, and China appears to have been selected as next in line to serve as bogeyman *du jour* — assuming that those of us with no access to fallout shelters are not vaporized in a nuclear holocaust first. While serving as the Democratic speaker of the House, Representative Nancy Pelosi, despite being a confirmed Faucista, did everything in her power to foment conflict with China by making a much-publicized and highly contentious visit in August 2022 to Taiwan, which appeared to be designed and timed precisely in order to antagonize China.[259]

The unanimous vote to declassify all documents relating to the COVID-19 virus origin was certainly not a salubrious sign that the U.S. republic is alive and well, and that we managed to dodge the dreaded totalitarian bullet. Indeed, shortly after the Twitter Files congressional hearing on March 9, 2023, in which journalists Matt Taibbi and Michael Shellenberger testified, many members of the House of Representatives voted against H.R. 140, the "Protecting Speech from Government Interference Act," which would prohibit the federal government from pressuring social media companies into muffling the voices of citizens exercising their right to free speech.[260] The act narrowly passed with a final vote of 219 to 206.

A great deal of the government-instigated censorship over the past three years related to the pandemic. Also noteworthy is that most of the same loyalist bloc of Democrats (201 representatives) voted on February 8, 2023, against lifting the illogical and unscientific vaccine mandate on foreign visitors attempting to enter the United States. The measure passed in the House (227 to 201) but was blocked by a Democrat in the Senate.[261] That requirement protects no one, while keeping families and friends apart, for the sole purpose, it seems, of punishing persons who declined to participate in the largest experimental trial of a novel medical device in human history. The only reason to uphold the mandate of a "vaccine" which prevents neither infection nor transmission is to support what has become the pathological predilection of U.S. presidents to issue executive orders. So what exactly is going on here?

The Twitter Files hearing spectacle made it clear that Congress has become so detached from the concerns of its constituents that fully half of its members are prepared to sign off on whatever the current administration wants to do, regardless of the likely consequences. As though programmed by whoever is running the Democratic Party show, surly representatives derided Taibbi and Shellenberger as "tinfoil hat conspiracy theorists" and "so-called journalists," in all likelihood because those soundbites would make excellent inquiry-shutdown headlines.[262] Predictably enough, the general response to the journalists' revelations by the networks has been a facile dismissal.

Given the anti-China march to war clearly underway, the networks may find hearings on the matter of virus origin more newsworthy than the sprawling Censorship-Industrial Complex (as Shellenberger termed it) — depending, of course, on what emerges. On March 8, 2023, witness Robert R. Redfield testified that the lab origin narrative was actively suppressed early in 2020 by Anthony Fauci and Francis Collins.[263] According to Dr. Redfield, a former director of the Centers for Disease Control and Prevention (CDC), Fauci and Collins, who were serving at the time as the head of the National Institute of Allergy and Infectious Diseases (NIAID) and the head of the National Institutes of Health (NIH), persuaded scientists who initially favored the gain-of-function hypothesis (as is documented in their email correspondence) to change their tune. The abrupt change in view was apparently effected during a conference call from which Redfield was excluded. Some months later, those same scientists were rewarded with millions of dollars of funding by the NIH.

Such suspicious machinations suggest that the concerned parties had something to hide, but shortly after Redfield's testimony, on March 16, 2023, author Kathryn J. Wu rushed to the rescue with a shiny new zoonotic theory about how it was not a pangolin and a bat kissing but a raccoon dog shedding virus (through sneezing?) near the wet market in Wuhan which gave rise to SARS-CoV-2.[264] One machination leads to another, and the publication of this novel theory in *The Atlantic* so soon after Redfield's testimony appears not to have been coincidental. (See the "yacht theory" of the Nord Stream sabotage for a similar example of *deus ex machina*.)

While inquiring minds mull over the raccoon dog hypothesis, the pharma-sponsored networks continue to invite recently retired Dr. Fauci to speak on their programs to bestow his latest words of wisdom upon the masses who came to view him as their savior throughout the Coronapocalypse. No matter that the outcomes for both virus and non-virus excess deaths in the United States were worse than nearly anywhere else in the world. Such Tertullian believers regularly commit the *post hoc ergo propter hoc* fallacy, thoroughly convinced as they are that, no matter how bad the outcomes were, they would have been much worse, if not for Dr. Anthony Fauci.

Even more remarkably, despite having co-authored a journal article published in January 2023 which plainly and unequivocally asserts that rapidly mutating viruses such as the flu and SARS-CoV-2 cannot, in principle, be controlled by vaccines (see Chapter 25), Fauci persists in making the rounds to chat with his chummy circuit of television talk show hosts, soberly explaining how "we" will be getting annual COVID-19 shots along with "our" flu shots. Notwithstanding the demonstrated mediocrity of both of those products, "we" will need to roll up our sleeves for the latest experimental elixirs apparently until the end of time, because, as Fauci puts it, "the virus is not going away." Nor is the common cold or the flu, neither of which, for the very same reasons elucidated in Fauci's own January 2023 publication, can be eliminated through the distribution of a vaccine. But habits die hard, and like a street corner pill pusher, Fauci cannot seem to refrain from peddling pharmaceutical wares to people who may or may not need them.

The evident plan is for new variants to be addressed through the creation of new "boosters," and Fauci can be depended upon by the product companies to use his perceived medical authority to promote a continual requirement of healthy persons to serve as experimental subjects for unnecessary remedies, which in some cases increase their risk of illness and organ damage. Difficult to believe though it may be, some universities continue to this day to require COVID-19 vaccination of their students, even bivalent booster shots already demonstrated to be of dubious efficacy. The COVID-19 shots, which offer healthy young persons a risk reduction on the order of 1%, at the same time significantly increase the risk among especially college-aged males of developing myocarditis and other heart conditions. Some private companies, too, persist in requiring vaccination as a condition of employment. In addition, a variety of arbitrary and nonsensical travel restrictions remain in place. When public health authorities make policy recommendations, managers and administrators assume that the prescribed measures are designed to protect the persons in their domain.

Recently leaked company documents made public by Project Veritas indicate that Pfizer was well aware, very early on, that their deceptively marketed, leaky vaccine had as serious adverse side effects heart inflammation (myocarditis) and related infirmities, including heart attacks and strokes.[265] When grilled on this topic by Senator Rand Paul in a recent hearing, Moderna CEO Stéphane Bancel (a newly minted billionaire thanks to the pandemic) professed ignorance of and indeed flatly denied this danger.[266] Senator Paul entered into the *Congressional Record* six peer-reviewed scientific studies, all of which conclude that myocarditis is a serious adverse effect particularly among males aged sixteen to twenty-four. But for the pharma giants, even deadly side effects are just a part of business as usual. Inured to the deleterious effects of their products on individual patients perfunctorily dismissed as *outliers*, the companies are driven only by the quest to sell more and more. If that requires marketers to hide or omit the truth, or executives such as Bancel to preserve a state of willful ignorance so that they can sleep at night, then so be it.

Even more significant than Bancel's professed ignorance of the dangers of vaccine-induced myocarditis was his answer to Senator Paul's inquiry regarding a conflict of interest created by Moderna's payment of $400 million of COVID-19 vaccine royalties to the NIH.[267] Bancel did not deny that giving government officials money might influence their judgment on where, when, and to whom to prescribe the very product from which they are profiting. Instead, he matter-of-factly replied, "This is for the government to decide."[268]

Therein lies the crux of the problem. In an oligarchic system such as our own, officials receive kickbacks for promoting the products of companies which reap hefty profits primarily as a result of government policies. (Strikingly, the first product ever brought to market by Moderna was the COVID-19 vaccine commissioned by the government.) In this way, a feedback loop is created whereby the interests of companies and bureaucrats are mutually supported, while the interests of the citizens whom elected officials supposedly serve are ignored. When institutions assess their own practices, there is no plausible scenario under which the very people who have allowed potentially compromising payments to take place would conclude that they were improper.

It is not without reason that Washington, D.C., is teeming with lobbyists for the pharmaceutical industry. Politicians who determine the laws of the land are showered with money by the Big Pharma giants. That money is then used in election campaigns, and the politicians, once reelected, become inclined to support the policies pushed by the lobbyists. Elected officials also appoint persons from the industry itself to government positions, for example, to head up the CDC, the NIH, the HHS (Department of Health and Human Services), and the VA (Veterans Administration).

In his analysis of the latest trove of Twitter company communications, Matt Taibbi has revealed how federal employees and their associated NGOs (sounds like a contradiction, I know) actively suppressed not only what they perceived to be disinformation, which in some cases was not, but also Tweets containing what *the censors themselves believed to be true information*, including reports of genuine vaccine injuries, on the grounds that such news would exacerbate vaccine hesitancy. The significance of this finding cannot be overstated.

There are two obvious ways in which to understand the censorship of what is believed to be true information in an effort to diminish vaccine hesitancy. The most charitable reading is that the censors embrace a quasi-utilitarian moral framework, according to which the right action maximizes the outcome of the greatest number. The pretext for censorship is, then, that more people would be harmed by the news than would be helped by it. Withholding the truth about the possibility of vaccine injury might persuade persons who would not otherwise have agreed to incur such a risk to undergo vaccination. But, at the same time, it would serve to encourage persons who needed the shots to get them. On balance, then, so the censor's reasoning goes, the news should be suppressed. While a few outliers may be harmed by the vaccines, many more persons will be saved than would be the case if the truth about adverse effects were allowed to be freely discussed among people still on the fence about whether or not to roll up their sleeves. This "benevolent" interpretation rests upon the assumption — now known to be false — that the COVID-19 "vaccines" are vaccines in the traditional sense, that is, capable of preventing infection and, most importantly from a public health perspective, transmission.

Censoring true stories of vaccine injuries negated informed consent by coercing compliance through deception. People were not only cajoled but in fact misled into taking the shots, which implies that those who were harmed can state without hyperbole that they were the victims of a government-perpetrated crime. What's more, the "greater good," or utilitarian pretext for maximizing vaccine uptake, was a fable all along, for the willingness of persons to undergo vaccination did not save anyone's grandparents, given that the leaky vaccines did not stop transmission. That some universities and private companies still require vaccination reveals that the erroneous belief that the COVID-19 vaccines prevent infection and transmission continues to guide the behavior of administrators and managers whose psyches were pommeled by a powerful propaganda campaign of fearmongering funded and perpetrated by coopted (or confused) government officials from 2020 to 2023.

Every bit as resilient as the lies used to garner support for the 2003 invasion of Iraq — that Saddam Hussein had WMD and was in cahoots with Osama bin Laden — the notion that "COVID-19 vaccines are safe and effective!" can be expected to remain firmly lodged in Branch Covidians' brains. Some of the most ardent vaccine advocates still occupy positions of government at the federal, state, and local level, and they will likely go to their graves muttering denunciations of what they have come to view as the evil *anti-vaxxers*. In reality, much of the vaccine hesitancy observed throughout the pandemic involved only a quite reasonable opposition to the notion that human beings should be forced to undergo an experimental treatment of which they have no need. It does not matter in the least what the consequences in the real world end up being, for "public health" drug pushers, just like warmongers, take refuge in their own good intentions and what they cast as the viciousness or stupidity of anyone who disagrees.

The second, far less charitable, but more plausible hypothesis for the censorship of true information about the new vaccines — especially given that they were never even tested in the initial trials to determine whether they effectively prevented transmission — is that the overarching concern, from the very beginning, was never to protect patients but to maximize the profits of the product companies. Such an interpretation, while admittedly unsavory, coheres well with the widespread and highly visible efforts to persuade pregnant women to undergo vaccination, even though members of that cohort were explicitly excluded from the trials used to secure Emergency Use Authorization (see Chapter 24). The same hypothesis would explain the incessant push to vaccinate small children for whom the risk of succumbing to the worst effects of COVID-19 has always been known to be minimal.

The primary reason why Matt Taibbi and Michael Shellenberger were treated at the Twitter Files hearing as disreputable by the Democratic representatives who questioned them is that they were reporting the very troubling fact that the U.S. government has in recent years invested no small amount of time, energy, and taxpayers' money in censoring citizens who dare to defy the official story of what is going on. That censorship and control of both social media and the mass media are carried out with the "good intentions" of protecting the people is just the latest version of the all-too-familiar line regularly recycled for every new military intervention abroad.

According to censors and warmakers, "We meant to do well!" That vacuous apology has paved the way for untold havoc wreaked on the people of other lands, but now we are facing the same delusional despotism draped in democratic robes at home as well. It is no coincidence that the advocates of censorship also stand ready to support any and every military intervention pitched in humanitarian terms, with no regard for the actual consequences on the ground. "Mistakes were made!" and "Stuff happens!" suffice in the minds of virtue-signaling "humanitarian interventionists" to wipe the moral slate clean.

As for the gain-of-function issue, because of Republicans' diaphanous desire to demonstrate that China was to blame for the millions of virus victims, we can expect the mystery to be solved sooner rather than later, even if for all the wrong reasons. For now, the jury is still out, but should the true story be far more disturbing than most of us imagined, the much-coveted war on China would make it a simple matter to obliterate the Wuhan Institute of Virology entirely, along with anyone in possession of potentially incriminatory evidence. Such a possibility may sound far-fetched, but lest anyone forget, in 1999, the U.S. military bombed the Chinese embassy in Belgrade based on CIA-sourced grid coordinates.

In the wake of the global upheaval from 2020 through 2023, the continual suggestion that there will be another global pandemic — for which, we have been repeatedly told, we must be prepared with a supranational response — perpetuates the fearmongering to continue to push shots on people who neither want nor need them. If the SARS-CoV-2 virus was in fact developed in a lab through gain-of-function research, and that is the *only* reason why it spread so quickly and killed so many people, then why does the director-general of the WHO (World Health Organization), Tedros Ghebreyesus, insist that we must prepare now for the next pandemic? One possibility is that he believes that gain-of-function research will continue on, and, therefore, another lab leak is inevitable, given human fallibility. But why should governments continue to fund gain-of-function research when the stakes are so high for humanity?

Herein lies yet another parallel (and overlap) with the military, for the analogous question can of course be asked of the incessant refinement of weapons of mass destruction, including bioweapons and, above all, nuclear arms. We know how dangerous such weapons are, and yet they continue to be developed and produced — and made even more lethal — on the pretext that if we do not create them first, then the evil enemy will beat us to them. As usual, however, the best explanation is the simplest explanation. Economic forces impel some people to push for the development of technology which will in fact endanger everyone else. The oligarchic crony capitalist scheme obviously governs the crafting of military policy, thanks to the revolving door of officers and corporate leaders. Former Raytheon board member Lloyd Austin now serves as the U.S. secretary of defense.

Profiteers, whether from the crony capitalist pharmaceutical industry or the crony capitalist military industry — and in some cases both — have by now coopted nearly every nook of the government, including most of the representatives elected by the people. As a result, it is nothing short of ludicrous to persist in the illusion that we live in a society even approximating a democratic republic. The elected officials have nearly all been persuaded to serve the winners of the crony capitalist system, both the military industry and the pharmaceutical industry, which explains why their political appointees do the same. No one should make the mistake of supposing that officials work for the people, for it is clear that they do not.

Bank bailouts are a third example of the very same phenomenon. How else can the support of such anti-capitalist corporate welfare by representatives who wish to eliminate entitlement programs for citizens be explained? As CEOs in not only the military and pharmaceutical industries but also finance have discovered, elected officials and the bureaucrats whom they appoint make the best profit multipliers of all because, so long as they wish to retain their positions, they will do everything in their power to shirk responsibility for past failures, and they will stand by their policies in the face of evidence that they were wrong or even disastrous. By establishing partnerships with government officials who possess the power not only to direct the allocation of public funds but also to render judgment on the wisdom of those allocations, CEOs of crony capitalist companies are able in this way to ensure ever-augmenting profits.

Many force multipliers are cultivated among the populace as well. The dynamics of narrative control by the government in evidence throughout the Twitter Files would seem to explain better than anything else why war continues to be cheered on by many people who do not even stand to profit, and despite the horrific outcomes of the obscene "War on Terror," which ended the lives of millions of people and terrorized and diminished the prospects of many times more. The U.S. military finally left Afghanistan after twenty years of claiming that the Taliban had to be defeated and democracy defended. Rather than regroup and assess the abject failure of the "War on Terror," the government has simply pretended that the Afghanistan fiasco never happened, pivoting smoothly to the next bogeyman, whether natural or manmade.

Throughout history, ordinary people, mere cogs in the machine, have made it possible for state atrocities to be perpetrated. The most plausible explanation of the censorship of true stories of vaccine injuries, as in the censorship of war crimes committed by the U.S. military, is that individuals convinced that they were doing the right thing (although they were laboring in a state of ignorance) served as force multipliers of the bad actors whose overarching aim was obviously to profit from crisis. Precisely as in the case of the war machine, in the recently forged pharma-government alliance, the road to hell is paved by useful stooges duped into supporting, under a spurious pretext of justice and morality, the forces driving the often megalomaniacal projects of elite oligarchs and their associated amoral mercenaries.

Appendix A:
The Great Barrington Declaration

As infectious disease epidemiologists and public health scientists we have grave concerns about the damaging physical and mental health impacts of the prevailing COVID-19 policies, and recommend an approach we call Focused Protection.

Coming from both the left and right, and around the world, we have devoted our careers to protecting people. Current lockdown policies are producing devastating effects on short- and long-term public health. The results (to name a few) include lower childhood vaccination rates, worsening cardiovascular disease outcomes, fewer cancer screenings and deteriorating mental health — leading to greater excess mortality in years to come, with the working class and younger members of society carrying the heaviest burden. Keeping students out of school is a grave injustice.

Keeping these measures in place until a vaccine is available will cause irreparable damage, with the underprivileged disproportionately harmed.

Fortunately, our understanding of the virus is growing. We know that vulnerability to death from COVID-19 is more than a thousand-fold higher in the old and infirm than the young. Indeed, for children, COVID-19 is less dangerous than many other harms, including influenza.

As immunity builds in the population, the risk of infection to all — including the vulnerable — falls. We know that all populations will eventually reach herd immunity — i.e., the point at which the rate of new infections is stable — and that this can be assisted by (but is not dependent upon) a vaccine. Our goal should therefore be to minimize mortality and social harm until we reach herd immunity.

The most compassionate approach that balances the risks and benefits of reaching herd immunity, is to allow those who are at minimal risk of death to live their lives normally to build up immunity to the virus through natural infection, while better protecting those who are at highest risk. We call this Focused Protection.

Adopting measures to protect the vulnerable should be the central aim of public health responses to COVID-19. By way of example, nursing homes should use staff with acquired immunity and perform frequent testing of other staff and all visitors. Staff rotation should be minimized. Retired people living at home should have groceries and other essentials delivered to their home. When possible, they should meet family members outside rather than inside. A comprehensive and detailed list of measures, including approaches to multigenerational households, can be implemented, and is well within the scope and capability of public health professionals.

Those who are not vulnerable should immediately be allowed to resume life as normal. Simple hygiene measures, such as hand washing and staying home when sick should be practiced by everyone to reduce the herd immunity threshold. Schools and universities should be open for in-person teaching.

Extracurricular activities, such as sports, should be resumed. Young low-risk adults should work normally, rather than from home. Restaurants and other businesses should open. Arts, music, sport and other cultural activities should resume. People who are more at risk may participate if they wish, while society as a whole enjoys the protection conferred upon the vulnerable by those who have built up herd immunity.

On October 4, 2020, this declaration was authored and signed in Great Barrington, United States, by:

Dr. Martin Kulldorff, professor of medicine at Harvard University, a biostatistician, and epidemiologist with expertise in detecting and monitoring infectious disease outbreaks and vaccine safety evaluations.
Dr. Sunetra Gupta, professor at Oxford University, an epidemiologist with expertise in immunology, vaccine development, and mathematical modeling of infectious diseases.
Dr. Jay Bhattacharya, professor at Stanford University Medical School, a physician, epidemiologist, health economist, and public health policy expert focusing on infectious diseases and vulnerable populations.

The complete list of signatories can be found at the Great Barrington Declaration website: gbdeclaration.org.

Appendix B: The Nuremberg Code

1. The voluntary consent of the human subject is absolutely essential. This means that the person involved should have legal capacity to give consent; should be so situated as to be able to exercise free power of choice, without the intervention of any element of force, fraud, deceit, duress, overreaching, or other ulterior form of constraint or coercion; and should have sufficient knowledge and comprehension of the elements of the subject matter involved as to enable him to make an understanding and enlightened decision. This latter element requires that before the acceptance of an affirmative decision by the experimental subject there should be made known to him the nature, duration, and purpose of the experiment; the method and means by which it is to be conducted; all inconveniences and hazards reasonably to be expected; and the effects upon his health or person which may possibly come from his participation in the experiment. The duty and responsibility for ascertaining the quality of the consent rests upon each individual who initiates, directs, or engages in the experiment. It is a personal duty and responsibility which may not be delegated to another with impunity.

2. The experiment should be such as to yield fruitful results for the good of society, unprocurable by other methods or means of study, and not random and unnecessary in nature.

3. The experiment should be so designed and based on the results of animal experimentation and a knowledge of the natural history of the disease or other problem under study that the anticipated results will justify the performance of the experiment.

4. The experiment should be so conducted as to avoid all unnecessary physical and mental suffering and injury.

5. No experiment should be conducted where there is an a priori reason to believe that death or disabling injury will occur; except, perhaps, in those experiments where the experimental physicians also serve as subjects.

6. The degree of risk to be taken should never exceed that determined by the humanitarian importance of the problem to be solved by the experiment.

7. Proper preparations should be made and adequate facilities provided to protect the experimental subject against even remote possibilities of injury, disability, or death.

8. The experiment should be conducted only by scientifically qualified persons. The highest degree of skill and care should be required through all stages of the experiment of those who conduct or engage in the experiment.

9. During the course of the experiment the human subject should be at liberty to bring the experiment to an end if he has reached the physical or mental state where continuation of the experiment seems to him to be impossible.

10. During the course of the experiment the scientist in charge must be prepared to terminate the experiment at any stage, if he has probable cause to believe, in the exercise of the good faith, superior skill and careful judgment required of him that a continuation of the experiment is likely to result in injury, disability, or death to the experimental subject.

Acknowledgements

I am grateful to Scott Horton for having welcomed me so warmly into the Libertarian Institute family, which has proven to be an oasis of intellectual activity in these rather arid times. I would also like to thank the various people who denounced me (in admittedly creative combinations) as an anti-vax, alt-right, fascist, QAnon, Trump supporter, none of which are in fact true. Their intent may have been to silence me, but it backfired, for I was motivated in part to forge on with my inquiries by the recognition that somehow people's brains were being infected by the media so as to drive them to the ludicrous conclusion that, because I am a critical thinker, I am *The Evil Enemy*. I won't name the names of those who unfriended, unfollowed, blocked, attempted to discredit, railed against, and shrieked at me. Needless to say, none of them will ever be reading this book anyway.

But there were also positive voices of encouragement along the way. I learned that my cousin Robert Jacks, Jr., and his wife, Susan, were very sympathetic with my concerns, and I had many fruitful and sanity-saving discussions about the Coronapocalypse, as early as February 2020, with Ulli Schwarzkopf, initially (in person) in Austria, and later over the Internet, while she was in Spain, and I was in either Austria, the U.K., or the United States. Ulli and her husband, Jim Dougherty, were also my gracious hosts throughout my five-month stay in the woods of Austria, where I was when all of this began. My hosts in London, artists Susan Stockwell and Michael Roberts, were extremely generous in offering to put me up for as long as I needed. We ended up sharing several dinners together, and I look forward to visiting them in France, where they have since relocated. Longstanding friends in the U.K., too, were always around to offer moral support and encourage me to return as soon as possible. Although I have a long list of good friends in the U.K., I feel that I must mention at least two of them: Sabina "Bee" Fisher-Jones and Lesley Clarke, for they not only welcomed me into their homes in the midst of the "global pandemic," but were always available to bounce ideas off of as this crisis continued to unfurl, seemingly with no end in sight. Stateside, I had a number of fruitful exchanges with Ajume Wingo, Mark Eckley, and Mike Church, among other inquiring minds, who may or may not appreciate seeing their names printed here. But you know who you are.

On the social media front, I received a fair amount of denunciation, but also plenty of positive feedback from persons whom I have never met in physical reality but now count among my virtual friends: Danielle Frenchie, Susan Lunde, David Sullivan, Joshua Holloway, Brad Pearce, Jale Richter, Luc de Broqueville, Ray Flash, Christos Karageorgos, and Magid Shihade all stand out as people who dared to interact with and even like my COVID posts when nearly everyone else appeared to delete them summarily. That my writings could not have been truly, intrinsically offensive would seem to be evidenced by the fact that I was never deplatformed by either Twitter or Facebook, despite the ever-lengthening series of my increasingly contrarian investigations.

Having now re-read all that I wrote, I find it somewhat amazing that anyone should have found my writings in any way objectionable, for most of these essays do not even rise to level of polemic. As the situation became progressively more dire, with very serious government initiatives not only to suppress dissent but even to inject unwilling subjects with experimental treatments, I occasionally veered into the territory of satire — so absurd had the situation become that humor seemed to be the only rational response.

I would like to thank all of my colleagues at the Libertarian Institute for their moral and intellectual support, and the book production team for their hard work on this project. Ben Parker, Mike Dworski, and Grant F. Smith turned my essays into a book. TheBumperSticker.com designed the cover.

The COVID-19 state of emergency in the United States ends officially today, on May 11, 2023, and I am happy to report that I am abroad once again, in Pontyclun, Wales.

Endnotes

[1] Kat Lay and Tom Calver, "Under-50s less likely to die from COVID-19 than from accident or injury," The Times, June 24, 2020, https://thetimes.co.uk/article/under-50s-less-likely-to-die-from-COVID-19-than-from-accident-or-injury-analysis-shows-9j6323qxt.
[2] "Global Deaths: This is how COVID-19 compares to other diseases," World Economic Forum, May 16, 2020, https://weforum.org/agenda/2020/05/how-many-people-die-each-day-COVID-19-coronavirus/.
[3] Laurie Calhoun. "Killing, Letting Die, and the Alleged Necessity of Military Intervention." *Peace and Conflict Studies* 8, no. 2 (2001). https://nsuworks.nova.edu/pcs/vol8/iss2/2/.
[4] Joseph Ax, "Bloomberg's ban on big sodas is unconstitutional: appeals court," Reuters, July 30, 2013, https://reuters.com/article/us-sodaban-lawsuit-idUSBRE96T0UT20130730.
[5] "The Top 10 Causes of Death," World Health Organization, December 9, 2020, https://who.int/news-room/fact-sheets/detail/the-top-10-causes-of-death.
[6] "Number of novel coronavirus (COVID-19) deaths worldwide, by country," Statista, https://statista.com/statistics/1093256/novel-coronavirus-2019ncov-deaths-worldwide-by-country/. Accessed August 21, 2020.
[7] "UK review into reporting COVID-19 deaths lowers toll by 5,000," Raidió Teilifís Éireann, August 12, 2020, https://rte.ie/news/2020/0812/1158865-england-covid-deaths/.
[8] Bernard Condon, Matt Sedensky, and Meghan Hoyer, "New York's true nursing home death toll cloaked in secrecy," AP News, August 11, 2020, https://apnews.com/article/virus-outbreak-ap-top-news-understanding-the-outbreak-new-york-andrew-cuomo-212ccd87924b6906053703a00514647f.
[9] Jon Miltimore, "Physicians Say Hospitals Are Pressuring ER Docs to List COVID-19 on Death Certificates. Here's Why," April 29, 2020, https://fee.org/articles/physicians-say-hospitals-are-pressuring-er-docs-to-list-COVID-19-on-death-certificates-here-s-why/.
[10] Jake Lahut, "NY Gov. Cuomo reportedly ordered over 4,300 recovering COVID-19 patients to be sent to nursing homes," *Business Insider*, May 22, 2020, https://businessinsider.com/cuomo-executive-order-4300-recovering-coronavirus-patients-ny-nursing-homes-2020-5?r=US&IR=T.
[11] Apoorva Mandavilli, "Your Coronavirus Test Is Positive. Maybe It Shouldn't Be," *New York Times*, August 29, 2020, https://nytimes.com/2020/08/29/health/coronavirus-testing.html.
[12] Richard Stevens, Richard Hobbs, Rafael Perera, and Jason Oke, "Should COVID-19 travel quarantine policy be based on apparent new case rates?" Centre for Evidence-Based Medicine, University of Oxford, https://cebm.net/2020/09/should-COVID-19-travel-quarantine-policy-be-based-on-apparent-new-case-rates/.

[13] Eriko Padron-Regalado. "Vaccines for SARS-CoV-2: Lessons from Other Coronavirus Strains," *Journal of Infectious Diseases & Therapy* 9, no. 2 (June 2020): 255–274. https://ncbi.nlm.nih.gov/pmc/articles/PMC7177048/.
[14] Naaman Zhou, "Victorian Bar criticises arrest of pregnant woman for Facebook lockdown protest post as 'disproportionate,'" *The Guardian*, September 3, 2020, https://theguardian.com/australia-news/2020/sep/03/victoria-police-arrested-pregnant-woman-facebook-post-zoe-buhler-australia-warn-lockdown-protesters.
[15] Wale Aliyu, "Northeastern dismisses 11 students caught partying in Boston hotel room, violating public health protocols," Boston 25 News, September 4, 2020, https://boston25news.com/news/local/northeastern-dismisses-11-students-gathering-boston-hotel-room-violating-public-health-protocols/HN7V2PFCX5A3ZAQINZMKE4NMPQ/.
[16] Emily Flitter, "'I Can't Keep Doing This': Small Business Owners Are Giving Up," *New York Times*, July 13, 2020, https://nytimes.com/2020/07/13/business/small-businesses-coronavirus.html.
[17] Leo Sher. "The Impact of the COVID-19 Pandemic on Suicide Rates." *QJM: An International Journal of Medicine* 113, no. 10. (June 2020). https://academic.oup.com/qjmed/article/113/10/707/5857612.
[18] "At least 13 dead as Peru police raid nightclub in Lima after Covid ban," *The Guardian*, August 23, 2020, https://theguardian.com/world/2020/aug/23/over-a-dozen-dead-as-peru-police-raid-nightclub-in-lima-over-covid-ban.
[19] "Flu Vaccine Now Required for all Massachusetts School Students Enrolled in Child Care Pre-School, K-12 and Post-Secondary Institutions," Massachusetts Department of Public Health, August 19, 2020, https://archives.lib.state.ma.us/bitstream/handle/2452/843141/on1249030866-2020-08-19.pdf?sequence=1&isAllowed=y.
[20] "CDC Seasonal Flu Effectiveness Studies," Centers for Disease Control and Prevention (CDC), https://cdc.gov/flu/vaccines-work/effectiveness-studies.htm.
[21] Laurie Calhoun, "Obedience to Authority: The Relevance of the Milgram Experiments in the Drone Age," The Drone Age, February 17, 2016, https://thedroneage.wordpress.com/2016/02/17/obedience-to-authority-the-relevance-of-the-milgram-experiments-in-the-drone-age/.
[22] Alex Turner-Cohen, "Coronavirus: WHO backflips on virus stance by condemning lockdowns," News.com.au, October 12, 2020, https://news.com.au/world/coronavirus/global/coronavirus-who-backflips-on-virus-stance-by-condemning-lockdowns/news-story/f2188f2aebff1b7b291b297731c3da74.
[23] April, Roach, "Ireland to be placed in second lockdown for six weeks as coronavirus cases rise," *Evening Standard*, October 19, 2020, https://standard.co.uk/news/world/ireland-coronavirus-lockdown-a4572206.html.
[24] Sam Blanchard, Ben Spencer, and Vanessa Chalmers, "Lockdowns DON'T work, study claims: Researchers say stay-at-home orders made no difference to coronavirus deaths around the world — but prior health levels DID," *Daily Mail*, July 23, 2020, https://dailymail.co.uk/news/article-8553929/Lockdowns-DONT-work-study-claims.html.

[25] "The Bullet and the Virus: Police brutality in Kenya's battle against coronavirus - BBC Africa Eye," BBC News Africa, June 15, 2020, https://youtube.com/watch?v=Eb3rV5mhpmQ.
[26] Susana Ferreira, "Portugal's radical drugs policy is working. Why hasn't the world copied it?" *The Guardian*, December 5, 2017, https://theguardian.com/news/2017/dec/05/portugals-radical-drugs-policy-is-working-why-hasnt-the-world-copied-it.
[27] Andrew Selsky, "Oregon leads the way in decriminalizing hard drugs," AP News, November 4, 2020, https://apnews.com/article/oregon-first-decriminalizing-hard-drugs-01edca37c776c9ea8bfd4afdd7a7a33e.
[28] "France, Germany Impose New Lockdown Measures as COVID-19 Cases Soar," VOA News, October 29, 2020, https://voanews.com/a/COVID-19-pandemic_france-germany-impose-new-lockdown-measures-COVID-19-cases-soar/6197721.html.
[29] Elena Surkova, Vladyslav Nikolayevskyy, and Francis Drobniewski. "False-positive COVID-19 results: hidden problems and costs." *The Lancet* 8, no. 12 (December 2020): 1167–1168. https://thelancet.com/journals/lanres/article/PIIS2213-2600(20)30453-7/fulltext.
[30] "CDC Seasonal Flu Effectiveness Studies," Centers for Disease Control and Prevention (CDC), https://cdc.gov/flu/vaccines-work/effectiveness-studies.htm.
[31] Diana Kwon, "The Promise of mRNA Vaccines," *The Scientist*, November 25, 2020, https://the-scientist.com/news-opinion/the-promise-of-mrna-vaccines-68202.
[32] Nick Paul Taylor, "AstraZeneca probes 'mistake' behind 90% COVID-19 vaccine efficacy," Fierce Biotech, November 24, 2020, https://fiercebiotech.com/biotech/astrazeneca-probes-mistake-behind-90-covid-vaccine-efficacy.
[33] Sonia Shah, *The Body Hunters: Testing New Drugs on the World's Poorest Patients* (New York: New Press, 2006), https://thenewpress.com/books/body-hunters.
[34] Lisa Schnirring, "Pfizer-BioNTech note 95% COVID vaccine efficacy, will apply for EUA," Center for Infectious Disease Research and Policy (CIDRAP), the University of Minnesota, November 18, 2020, https://cidrap.umn.edu/news-perspective/2020/11/pfizer-biontech-note-95-covid-vaccine-efficacy-will-apply-eua.
[35] Robert Whitaker, "Do Antidepressants Work? A People's Review of the Evidence," Mad in America, March 11, 2018, https://madinamerica.com/2018/03/do-antidepressants-work-a-peoples-review-of-the-evidence/.
[36] Donald L. Luskin, "The Failed Experiment of COVID Lockdowns," *Wall Street Journal*, September 1, 2020, https://wsj.com/articles/the-failed-experiment-of-covid-lockdowns-11599000890.
[37] "Covid Vaccination will be required to fly, says Qantas chief," BBC News, November 23, 2020, https://bbc.com/news/world-australia-55048438.
[38] Andrew C. McCarthy, "For Thanksgiving, the Supreme Court upholds religious liberty," *The Hill*, November 28, 2020, https://thehill.com/opinion/judiciary/527773-for-thanksgiving-the-supreme-court-upholds-religious-liberty/.

[39] "Brazil's Bolsonaro says he will not take coronavirus vaccine," Reuters, November 26, 2020, https://reuters.com/article/us-brazil-bolsonaro-vaccine/brazils-bolsonaro-says-he-will-not-take-coronavirus-vaccine-idUSKBN28704L.
[40] Avery Hartmans, "Elon Musk says he and his family won't get a coronavirus vaccine when it becomes available," *Business Insider*, September 28, 2020, https://businessinsider.com/elon-musk-and-kids-wont-get-coronavirus-vaccine-2020-9.
[41] Hannah Arendt, *Eichmann in Jerusalem: A Report on the Banality of Evil* (New York: Penguin Classics, 2006), https://penguinrandomhouse.com/books/320983/eichmann-in-jerusalem-by-hannah-arendt/.
[42] Max Abrahms, "Don't Give Domestic Extremists the 'Post-9/11 Treatment,'" *Reason*, January 22, 2021, https://reason.com/2021/01/22/dont-give-domestic-extremists-the-post-9-11-treatment/.
[43] Martin Kulldorff, Sunetra Gupta, Jay Bhattacharya, et al., "Great Barrington Declaration," October 4, 2020, https://gbdeclaration.org/
[44] Children's Health Defense, https://childrenshealthdefense.org/.
[45] "Think of others — get a COVID shot, says UK's Queen Elizabeth," Reuters, February 26, 2021, https://reuters.com/article/us-britain-royals-queen/dont-be-selfish-get-a-covid-shot-says-uks-queen-elizabeth-idUSKBN2AQ0U1.
[46] Laurie Calhoun, "British Drone Strike Targets in the Light of the Chilcot Report," The Drone Age, August 22, 2016, https://thedroneage.wordpress.com/2016/08/22/british-drone-strike-targets-in-the-light-of-the-chilcot-report/.
[47] Suzanne Rowan Kelleher, "Why Vaccine Passports are 'Inevitable,' Explained by Tony Blair," *Forbes*, February 13, 2021, https://forbes.com/sites/suzannerowankelleher/2021/02/13/why-vaccine-passports-are-inevitable-explained-by-tony-blair/?sh=527ec18041d6.
[48] Nicole Chenoweth, "HANK-ING IN THERE: Tom Hanks admits he still feels 'blah' but has 'no fever' during coronavirus battle after being released," *The U.S. Sun*, March 17, 2020, https://the-sun.com/entertainment/552484/tom-hanks-coronavirus-blah-fever-released-hospital/.
[49] Matthew J. Belvedere, "Bill Gates: My 'best investment' turned $10 billion into $200 billion worth of economic benefit," CNBC, January 23, 2019, https://cnbc.com/2019/01/23/bill-gates-turns-10-billion-into-200-billion-worth-of-economic-benefit.html.
[50] "Tuskegee Syphilis Study," Wikipedia, https://en.wikipedia.org/wiki/Tuskegee_Syphilis_Study. Accessed April 2, 2021.
[51] "Eunice Rivers Laurie," Wikipedia, https://en.wikipedia.org/wiki/Eunice_Rivers_Laurie. Accessed April 2, 2021.
[52] "Thalidomide," Wikipedia, https://en.wikipedia.org/wiki/Thalidomide. Accessed April 2, 2021.
[53] "Immunization: The Basics" (Archive link), Centers for Disease Control and Prevention, http://web.archive.org/web/20210826113846/https://cdc.gov/vaccines/vac-gen/imz-basics.htm. Last modified May 17, 2018.

[54] "About us: Our Story," Moderna, Inc., https://modernatx.com/about-us/our-story. Accessed April 2, 2021.
[55] MacKenzie Sigalos, "You can't sue Pfizer or Moderna if you have severe Covid vaccine side effects. The government likely won't compensate you for damages either," CNBC, December 23, 2020, https://cnbc.com/2020/12/16/covid-vaccine-side-effects-compensation-lawsuit.html.
[56] "Drug Approvals — From Invention to Market… A 12-Year Trip," July 14, 1999, https://medicinenet.com/script/main/art.asp?articlekey=9877.
[57] Alex N. Livingston and T. Joseph Mattingly II. "Drug and medical device product failures and the stability of the pharmaceutical supply chain," *Journal of the American Pharmacists Association* 61, no. 1 (January/February 2021): 119–122. https://ncbi.nlm.nih.gov/pmc/articles/PMC7395820/.
[58] "10 Biggest Pharmaceutical Settlements in History," Enjuris, June 2020, https://enjuris.com/blog/resources/largest-pharmaceutical-settlements-lawsuits/.
[59] "Pfizer-BioNTech Fact Sheets," Food and Drug Administration, March 16, 2023, https://fda.gov/emergency-preparedness-and-response/coronavirus-disease-2019-COVID-19/pfizer-biontech-COVID-19-vaccines#additional.
[60] "Moderna COVID-19 Vaccine EUA Fact Sheet for Recipients and Caregivers," Food and Drug Administration, August 31, 2022, https://fda.gov/media/144638/download.
[61] Connor Boyd, "Revealed: Average age of COVID-19 victims is OLDER than life expectancy in Scotland as stark figures show 'it is predominantly a disease that strikes the elderly,'" *Daily Mail*, July 21, 2020, https://dailymail.co.uk/news/article-8470843/The-average-COVID-19-victim-OLDER-age-people-usually-die-Scotland.html.
[62] Lauren Fox, Sarah Fortinsky, Kristin Wilson, and Ali Zaslav, "Inside why all lawmakers still aren't vaccinated after months of access to shots on the Hill," *CNN Politics*, March 19, 2021, https://cnn.com/2021/03/19/politics/lawmakers-not-all-vaccinated-capitol-hill/index.html.
[63] Xiao-Lin Jiang, Guo-Lin Wang, Xiang-Na Zhao, Fei-Hu Yan, Lin Yao, Zeng-Qiang Kou, Sheng-Xiang Ji, Xiao-Li Zhang, Cun-Bao Li, Li-Jun Duan, Yan Li, Yu-Wen Zhang, Qing Duan, Tie-Cheng Wang, En-Tao Li, Xiao Wei, Qing-Yang Wang, Xue-Feng Wang, Wei-Yang Sun, Yu-Wei Gao, Dian-Min Kang, Ji-Yan Zhang, and Mai-Juan Ma. "Lasting antibody and T-cell responses to SARS-CoV-2 in COVID-19 patients three months after infection," *Nature Communications* 12, no. 897 (February 2021). https://nature.com/articles/s41467-021-21155-x.
[64] Bojan Pancevski, "Scientists Say They Found Cause of Rare Blood Clotting Linked to AstraZeneca Vaccine," *Wall Street Journal*, March 19, 2021, https://wsj.com/articles/scientists-say-they-found-cause-of-blood-clotting-linked-to-astrazeneca-vaccine-11616169108.
[65] "NEW COVID-19 Vaccine Offer | ONE WEEK ONLY!" Krispy Kreme, Inc., March 23, 2021, https://krispykreme.com/promos/vaccineoffer (Archive link: https://web.archive.org/web/20210323234831/https://krispykreme.com/promos/vaccineoffer).
[66] John Tamny, "The Truth About the Biden Tax Plan," May 11, 2021, https://libertarianinstitute.org/articles/the-truth-about-the-biden-tax-plan/.

[67] Brittany Shammas, "Pelosi faces backlash after thanking George Floyd for 'sacrificing your life for justice,'" *Washington Post*, April 21, 2021, https://washingtonpost.com/politics/2021/04/21/nancy-pelosi-george-floyd/.
[68] Laurie Calhoun, "The Jig is Up: Just War Theory Can No Longer Be Used as a Cover for State Policies of Mass Homicide," May 3, 2016, https://antiwar.com/blog/2016/05/03/the-jig-is-up-just-war-theory-can-no-longer-be-used-as-a-cover-for-state-policies-of-mass-homicide/.
[69] Laurie Calhoun, "'We Murdered Some Folks': How Self-Styled Drone Warrior U.S. President Barack Obama Normalized War Crimes (Part 3)," The Drone Age, July 11, 2016, https://thedroneage.wordpress.com/2016/07/11/we-murdered-some-folks-how-self-styled-drone-warrior-us-president-barack-obama-normalized-war-crimes-part-3/.
[70] "Military Spending in the United States," National Priorities Project, Institute for Policy Studies, https://nationalpriorities.org/campaigns/military-spending-united-states/. Accessed May 13, 2021.
[71] "Ponzi Scheme," U.S. Securities and Exchange Commission, https://investor.gov/protect-your-investments/fraud/types-fraud/ponzi-scheme. Accessed June 21, 2021.
[72] Scott Horton, *Enough Already: Time to End the War on Terrorism* (Austin: The Libertarian Institute, 2021), https://libertarianinstitute.org/books/enough-already-time-to-end-the-war-on-terrorism/.
[73] "U.S. National Debt Clock," USDebtClock.org, https://usdebtclock.org/.
[74] "About Halliburton," Halliburton Watch, https://halliburtonwatch.org/about_hal/logcap.html. Accessed June 21, 2021.
[75] "Number of People Taking Psychiatric Drugs in the United States (Data extracted from TPT (*Total Patient Tracker*) database January 2021)," Citizens Commission on Human Rights International, https://cchrint.org/psychiatric-drugs/people-taking-psychiatric-drugs/. Accessed June 21, 2021.
[76] Nicole Lyn Pesce, "Anti-anxiety medication prescriptions have spiked 34% during the coronavirus pandemic," Market Watch, May 26, 2020, https://marketwatch.com/story/anti-anxiety-medication-prescriptions-have-spiked-34-during-the-coronavirus-pandemic-2020-04-16.
[77] "The Drug Overdose Epidemic: Behind the Numbers," Centers for Disease Control and Prevention, June 1, 2022, https://cdc.gov/opioids/data/index.html.
[78] Gerald Posner, *Pharma: Greed, Lies, and the Poisoning of America* (New York: Simon & Schuster, 2020), https://simonandschuster.com/books/Pharma/Gerald-Posner/9781501152030.
[79] Lev Facher and Kaitlyn Bartley, "Prescription Politics: Pharma is showering Congress with cash, even as drug makers race to fight the coronavirus," *STAT News*, August 10, 2020, https://statnews.com/feature/prescription-politics/prescription-politics/.
[80] Martha Rosenberg, "The Rise and Fall of the Blockbuster Antipsychotic Seroquel," Center for Health Journalism, USC-Annenberg, November 26, 2015, https://centerforhealthjournalism.org/fellowships/projects/rise-and-fall-blockbuster-antipsychotic-seroquel. (Archive link: https://web.archive.org/web/20210627050700/https://centerforhealthjournalism.org/fellowships/projects/rise-and-fall-blockbuster-antipsychotic-seroquel).

[81] Pierre Kory, MD; Gianfranco Umberto Meduri, MD; Joseph Varon, MD; Jose Iglesias, DO; and Paul E. Marik, MD. "Review of the Emerging Evidence Demonstrating the Efficacy of Ivermectin in the Prophylaxis and Treatment of COVID-19." *American Journal of Therapeutics* 28, no. 3 (May/June 2021): 299–318. https://journals.lww.com/americantherapeutics/fulltext/2021/06000/review_of_the_emerging_evidence_demonstrating_the.4.aspx.
[82] Robin Erb, "Henry Ford study on hydroxychloroquine for COVID quietly shut down," *Bridge Michigan*, January 11, 2021, https://bridgemi.com/michigan-health-watch/henry-ford-study-hydroxychloroquine-covid-quietly-shut-down.
[83] "Pfizer-BioNTech Fact Sheets."
[84] "Moderna COVID-19 Vaccine EUA Fact Sheet for Recipients and Caregivers," Food and Drug Administration, August 31, 2022, https://fda.gov/media/144638/download.
[85] Noah Weiland, Denise Grady, and David E. Sanger, "Pfizer Gets $1.95 Billion to Produce Coronavirus Vaccine by Year's End," *New York Times*, July 22, 2020, https://nytimes.com/2020/07/22/us/politics/pfizer-coronavirus-vaccine.html.
[86] "President Biden Announces Historic Vaccine Donation: Half a Billion Pfizer Vaccines to the World's Lowest-Income Nations," June 10, 2021, https://whitehouse.gov/briefing-room/statements-releases/2021/06/10/fact-sheet-president-biden-announces-historic-vaccine-donation-half-a-billion-pfizer-vaccines-to-the-worlds-lowest-income-nations/.
[87] Piero Olliaro, Els Torreele, and Michel Vaillant. "COVID-19 Vaccine Efficacy and Effectiveness — The Elephant (Not) in the Room." *The Lancet* 2, no. 7 (July 2021): 279–280. https://thelancet.com/journals/lanmic/article/PIIS2666-5247(21)00069-0/fulltext.
[88] "COVID-19 reinfection tracker," BNO News, August 28, 2020, https://bnonews.com/index.php/2020/08/COVID-19-reinfection-tracker/.
[89] Ewen Callaway, "Had COVID? You'll probably make antibodies for a lifetime," *Nature*, May 26, 2021, https://nature.com/articles/d41586-021-01442-9.
[90] Sanchari Sinha Dutta, Ph.D., "No point vaccinating those who've had COVID-19: Cleveland Clinic Study Suggests," *Medical News*, June 8, 2021, https://news-medical.net/news/20210608/No-point-vaccinating-those-whoe28099ve-had-COVID-19-Findings-of-Cleveland-Clinic-study.aspx.
[91] Timothy Annett, "Pfizer CEO Bourla's Pay Climbed 17% to $21 Million in 2020," Bloomberg News, March 12, 2021, https://bnnbloomberg.ca/pfizer-ceo-bourla-s-pay-climbed-17-to-21-million-in-2020-1.1576267.
[92] Giacomo Tognini, "Moderna CEO Stéphane Bancel Becomes a Billionaire as Stock Jumps on Coronavirus Vaccine News," *Forbes*, April 3, 2020, https://forbes.com/sites/giacomotognini/2020/04/03/moderna-ceo-stphane-bancel-becomes-a-billionaire-as-stock-jumps-on-coronavirus-vaccine-news/?sh=71dff8bc5bf3.
[93] Sam Husseini, "Peter Daszak's EcoHealth Alliance Has Hidden Almost $40 Million in Pentagon Funding and Militarized Pandemic Science," *Independent Science News*, December 16, 2020, https://independentsciencenews.org/news/peter-daszaks-ecohealth-alliance-has-hidden-almost-40-million-in-pentagon-funding/.
[94] "Spot the Lockdowns," COVID Charts Quiz, https://covidchartsquiz.com/lockdowns.

[95] Laurie Calhoun. "Killing, Letting Die, and the Alleged Necessity of Military Intervention." *Peace and Conflict Studies* 8, no. 2 (2001). https://nsuworks.nova.edu/pcs/vol8/iss2/2/.
[96] Scott Horton, *Enough Already: Time to End the War on Terrorism* (Austin: The Libertarian Institute, 2021), https://libertarianinstitute.org/books/enough-already-time-to-end-the-war-on-terrorism/.
[97] Laurie Calhoun, *War and Delusion: A Critical Examination* (New York: Palgrave Macmillan, 2013), https://link.springer.com/book/10.1057/9781137294630.
[98] Lee Black, JD, LLM. "Informed Consent in the Military: The Anthrax Vaccination Case." *AMA Journal of Ethics* 9, no. 10 (October 2007): 698–792. https://journalofethics.ama-assn.org/article/informed-consent-military-anthrax-vaccination-case/2007-10.
[99] "Vaccine Adverse Event Reporting System (VAERS)," Health and Human Services (HHS), https://vaers.hhs.gov/.
[100] Mark Lungariello, "Ohio judge requires COVID vaccines as part of probation," *New York Post*, July 1, 2021, https://nypost.com/2021/07/01/ohio-judge-requires-covid-vaccines-as-part-of-probation/.
[101] Constantin Gouvy and Angela Charlton, "French rush to get vaccinated after president's warning," AP News, July 13, 2021, https://apnews.com/article/europe-business-lifestyle-health-travel-1d10271c4f1617521892d49d83b773ad.
[102] Michael D. Shear and Noah Weiland, "Biden Calls for Door-to-Door Vaccine Push; Experts Say More Is Needed," *New York Times*, July 6, 2021, https://nytimes.com/2021/07/06/us/politics/biden-vaccines.html.
[103] Piero Olliaro, Els Torreele, and Michel Vaillant. "COVID-19 Vaccine Efficacy and Effectiveness — The Elephant (Not) in the Room." *The Lancet* 2, no. 7 (July 2021): 279–280. https://thelancet.com/journals/lanmic/article/PIIS2666-5247(21)00069-0/fulltext.
[104] "Collateral Murder," WikiLeaks, April 5, 2010, https://collateralmurder.wikileaks.org/.
[105] Laurie Calhoun, "The Drone Program Whistleblower Problem," August 2, 2021, https://libertarianinstitute.org/articles/the-drone-program-whistleblower-problem/.
[106] Glenn Greenwald, "A Court Ruled Rachel Maddow's Viewers Know She's Not Offering Facts," *Scheer Post*, June 22, 2021, https://scheerpost.com/2021/06/22/a-court-ruled-rachel-maddows-viewers-know-shes-not-offering-facts/.
[107] Rachel Maddow, *Drift: The Unmooring of American Military Power* (New York: Random House, 2012), https://penguinrandomhouse.com/books/105954/drift-by-rachel-maddow/.
[108] "Stanley A. McChrystal," Wikipedia, https://en.wikipedia.org/wiki/Stanley_A._McChrystal#Rolling_Stone_article_and_resignation. Accessed August 24, 2021.
[109] Laurie Calhoun, "'We Murdered Some Folks': How Self-Styled Drone Warrior U.S. President Barack Obama Normalized War Crimes (Part 3)," The Drone Age, July 11, 2016, https://thedroneage.wordpress.com/2016/07/11/we-murdered-some-folks-how-self-styled-drone-warrior-us-president-barack-obama-normalized-war-crimes-part-3/.

[110] José María Irujo, "Spanish firm that spied on Julian Assange tried to find out if he fathered a child at Ecuadorian Embassy," *El País*, April 15, 2020, https://english.elpais.com/international/2020-04-15/spanish-firm-that-spied-on-julian-assange-tried-to-find-out-if-he-fathered-a-child-at-ecuadorian-embassy.html.
[111] Brian McGleenon, "US spies 'plotted to poison Julian Assange and make it look like an accident,'" *Daily Express*, February 25, 2020, https://express.co.uk/news/world/1247248/us-plot-julian-assange-extradition-trial-cia-secret-documents.
[112] Bjartmar Oddur Þeyr Alexandersson and Gunnar Hrafn Jónsson, "Key witness in Assange case admits to lies in indictment," *Stundin* (now *Heimildin*), June 26, 2021, https://stundin.is/grein/13627/.
[113] "Afghan War Diary" (archive), WikiLeaks, https://wikileaks.org/wiki/Afghan_War_Diary,_2004-2010.
[114] "Baghdad War Diary" (archive), WikiLeaks, https://wikileaks.org/irq/.
[115] Emma Colton, "Psaki says administration is working with Facebook to limit misinformation," Fox Business, July 16, 2021, https://foxbusiness.com/politics/white-house-facebook-vaccine-misinformation.
[116] Jacob Jarvis, "Fact Check: Did Donald Trump Suggest People Inject Poison to Cure COVID?" *Newsweek*, August 16, 2021, https://newsweek.com/fact-check-did-donald-trump-suggest-people-inject-poison-cure-covid-1619105.
[117] Joshua Keating, "Why the U.S. Government Took Down Dozens of Iranian Websites This Week," *Slate*, June 24, 2021, https://slate.com/technology/2021/06/presstv-iranian-websites-justice-department-seizure.html.
[118] Alex Hern, "'YouTube Islamist' Anwar al-Awlaki videos removed in extremism clampdown," *The Guardian*, November 13, 2017, https://theguardian.com/technology/2017/nov/13/youtube-islamist-anwar-al-awlaki-videos-removed-google-extremism-clampdown.
[119] Laurie Calhoun, "Do the Math: How Self-Styled Drone Warrior U.S. President Barack Obama Normalized War Crimes (Part 1)," The Drone Age, July 4, 2016, https://thedroneage.wordpress.com/2016/07/04/do-the-math-part-1-of-how-self-styled-drone-warrior-us-president-barack-obama-normalized-war-crimes/.
[120] "Pfizer-BioNTech Fact Sheets."
[121] "Moderna COVID-19 Vaccine EUA Fact Sheet for Recipients and Caregivers," Food and Drug Administration, August 31, 2022, https://fda.gov/media/144638/download.
[122] "Justice Department Announces Largest Healthcare Fraud Settlement in Its History," U.S. Department of Justice, September 2, 2009, https://justice.gov/opa/pr/justice-department-announces-largest-health-care-fraud-settlement-its-history.
[123] "Chantix linked to Heart Attack, Stroke, Suicide, Depression, and Unexplained Aggression," Levin Simes, LLP, July 9, 2020, https://levinsimes.com/blog/chantix-linked-to-heart-attack-stroke-suicide-depression-and-unexplained-aggression/ (Archive link: https://web.archive.org/web/20211203082402/https://levinsimes.com/blog/chantix-linked-to-heart-attack-stroke-suicide-depression-and-unexplained-aggression/).

[124] Nicole Acevedo, "Pfizer recalls all lots of anti-smoking drug Chantix over carcinogen presence," NBC News, September 18, 2021, https://nbcnews.com/news/us-news/pfizer-recalls-all-lots-anti-smoking-drug-chantix-over-carcinogen-n1279503.
[125] Tiffany Hsu, "Black women's group sues Johnson & Johnson over talc baby powder," *New York Times*, July 27, 2021, https://nytimes.com/2021/07/27/business/johnson-baby-powder-black-women.html.
[126] "AstraZeneca vaccine: Denmark stops rollout completely," BBC News, April 14, 2021, https://bbc.com/news/world-europe-56744474.
[127] "Pharmaceutical Giant AstraZeneca to Pay $520 Million for Off-label Drug Marketing," U.S. Department of Justice, April 27, 2010, https://justice.gov/opa/pr/pharmaceutical-giant-astrazeneca-pay-520-million-label-drug-marketing.
[128] Matthew Perrone, "Deaths raise questions on drug given to sleepless vets," NBC News, August 30, 2010, https://nbcnews.com/health/health-news/deaths-raise-questions-drug-given-sleepless-vets-flna1c9477171.
[129] John Horgan, "Are Antidepressants Just Placebos with Side Effects?" *Scientific American*, July 12, 2011, https://blogs.scientificamerican.com/cross-check/are-antidepressants-just-placebos-with-side-effects/.
[130] "DARPA Awards Moderna up to $56 Million to Enable Small-Scale, Rapid Mobile Manufacturing of Nucleic Acid Vaccines and Therapeutics," Moderna, Inc., October 8, 2020, https://investors.modernatx.com/news/news-details/2020/DARPA-Awards-Moderna-up-to-56-Million-to-Enable-Small-Scale-Rapid-Mobile-Manufacturing-of-Nucleic-Acid-Vaccines-and-Therapeutics/default.aspx.
[131] Marty Makary, "Natural Immunity to COVID is Powerful. Policymakers seem afraid to say so," *Washington Post*, September 15, 2021, https://washingtonpost.com/outlook/2021/09/15/natural-immunity-vaccine-mandate/.
[132] Ian Sample, "Boys more at risk from Pfizer jab side effect than Covid, suggests study," *The Guardian*, September 10, 2021, https://theguardian.com/world/2021/sep/10/boys-more-at-risk-from-pfizer-jab-side-effect-than-covid-suggests-study.
[133] "Vaccine Adverse Event Reporting System (VAERS)," Health and Human Services (HHS), https://vaers.hhs.gov/.
[134] "Public Readiness and Preparedness (PREP) Act," Health and Human Services (HHS), December 2005, https://aspr.hhs.gov/legal/PREPact/Pages/default.aspx.
[135] Glenn Greenwald, "Pierre Omidyar's Financing of the Facebook 'Whistleblower' Campaign Reveals a Great Deal," *Glenn Greenwald | Substack*, October 25, 2021, https://greenwald.substack.com/p/pierre-omidyars-financing-of-the.
[136] Sophie Mellor, "Mark Zuckerberg should quit Facebook, whistleblower Frances Haugen says," *Fortune*, November 1, 2021, https://fortune.com/2021/11/01/mark-zuckerberg-should-quit-facebook-whistleblower-frances-haugen-says/.

[137] Laurie Calhoun, "A Fitting Flourish on a 20-Year Killing Spree," September 13, 2021, https://libertarianinstitute.org/articles/a-fitting-flourish-on-a-20-year-killing-spree/.
[138] Brandon Bryant (archive), The Drone Age, https://thedroneage.wordpress.com/tag/brandon-bryant/.
[139] Laurie Calhoun, "Chew 'Em Up and Spit 'Em Out: The Drone Operator Edition," The Drone Age, December 17, 2015, https://thedroneage.wordpress.com/2015/12/17/chew-em-up-and-spit-em-out-the-drone-operator-edition/.
[140] Laurie Calhoun, "The Drone Program Whistleblower Problem," August 2, 2021, https://libertarianinstitute.org/articles/the-drone-program-whistleblower-problem/.
[141] "The Drone Papers" (archive), *The Intercept*, https://theintercept.com/drone-papers/.
[142] Jeremy Scahill, *The Assassination Complex: Inside the Government's Secret Drone Warfare Program* (New York: Simon & Schuster, 2016), https://simonandschuster.com/books/The-Assassination-Complex/Jeremy-Scahill/9781501144141.
[143] Laurie Calhoun, *War and Delusion: A Critical Examination* (New York: Palgrave Macmillan, 2013), https://link.springer.com/book/10.1057/9781137294630.
[144] Laurie Calhoun, *We Kill Because We Can: From Soldiering to Assassination in the Drone Age* (London: Zed Books Ltd., 2015), https://bloomsbury.com/us/we-kill-because-we-can-9781783605491/.
[145] Laurie Calhoun, "A Fitting Flourish on a 20-Year Killing Spree," September 13, 2021, https://libertarianinstitute.org/articles/a-fitting-flourish-on-a-20-year-killing-spree/.
[146] "Teenagers from remote NT community arrested after escape from Howard Springs COVID Facility," Australian Broadcasting Corporation, November 30, 2021, https://abc.net.au/news/2021-12-01/multiple-people-escape-howard-springs-quarantine-facility-darwin/100663994.
[147] Scott Horton, *Fool's Errand: Time to End the War in Afghanistan* (Austin: The Libertarian Institute, 2017), https://foolserrand.us/.
[148] Oliver Noyan, "Austria considers €7,200 fine for unvaccinated," Euractiv, November 29, 2021, https://euractiv.com/section/politics/short_news/austria-considers-e7200-fine-for-unvaccinated/.
[149] "Drug Maker Pfizer Agrees to Pay $23.85 Million to Resolve False Claims Act Liability for Paying Kickbacks," U.S. Department of Justice, May 24, 2018, https://justice.gov/opa/pr/drug-maker-pfizer-agrees-pay-2385-million-resolve-false-claims-act-liability-paying-kickbacks.
[150] Joseph Biden, "Remarks by President Biden on Fighting the COVID-19 Pandemic," September 9, 2021, https://whitehouse.gov/briefing-room/speeches-remarks/2021/09/09/remarks-by-president-biden-on-fighting-the-COVID-19-pandemic-3/.
[151] Ian Sample, "Boys more at risk from Pfizer jab side effect than Covid, suggests study," *The Guardian*, September 10, 2021, https://theguardian.com/world/2021/sep/10/boys-more-at-risk-from-pfizer-jab-side-effect-than-covid-suggests-study.

[152] Rob Picheta, "UK to offer booster shots to all adults, just three months after their second dose," *CNN World*, November 29, 2021, https://cnn.com/2021/11/29/uk/uk-booster-vaccine-expansion-omicron-gbr-intl/index.html.
[153] Jane Dalton, "Charity warns of 50,000 'missing' cancer cases with backlog 'still to hit NHS,'" *The Independent*, November 26, 2021, https://independent.co.uk/news/health/cancer-treatment-nhs-macmillan-missing-b1964470.html.
[154] Ben Goldacre, *Bad Pharma: How Drug Companies Mislead Doctors and Harm Patients* (New York: Faber and Faber, Inc., 2014), https://us.macmillan.com/books/9780865478060.
[155] "Industry Totals (Pharmaceuticals/Health Products): 2020 Presidential Race," OpenSecrets.org, https://opensecrets.org/2020-presidential-race/industry-totals?highlight=y&ind=H04&src=a. Accessed February 1, 2022.
[156] "Biden Administration to Begin Distributing At-Home, Rapid COVID-19 Tests to Americans for Free," January 14, 2022, https://whitehouse.gov/briefing-room/statements-releases/2022/01/14/fact-sheet-the-biden-administration-to-begin-distributing-at-home-rapid-COVID-19-tests-to-americans-for-free/.
[157] Jeremy Diamond and Paul LeBlanc, "Biden administration to distribute 400 million N95 masks to the public for free," *CNN Politics*, January 19, 2022, https://cnn.com/2022/01/19/politics/n95-masks-biden-administration-COVID-19/index.html.
[158] Spencer Kimball, "Pfizer CEO says omicron vaccine will be ready in March," CNBC, January 10, 2022, https://cnbc.com/2022/01/10/covid-vaccine-pfizer-ceo-says-omicron-vaccine-will-be-ready-in-march.html.
[159] Laurie Calhoun. "The Silencing of Soldiers." *The Independent Review* 16, no. 2 (Fall 2011): pp. 247–270. https://independent.org/pdf/tir/tir_16_02_6_calhoun.pdf.
[160] Jon Cohen, "Why is the flu vaccine so mediocre?" *Science*, September 22, 2017, https://science.org/doi/10.1126/science.357.6357.1222.
[161] "PREP Act Immunity from Liability for COVID-19 Vaccinators," April 13, 2021, https://phe.gov/emergency/events/COVID19/COVIDVaccinators/Pages/PREP-Act-Immunity-from-Liability-for-COVID-19-Vaccinators.aspx.
[162] Piero Olliaro, Els Torreele, and Michel Vaillant. "COVID-19 Vaccine Efficacy and Effectiveness — The Elephant (Not) in the Room." *The Lancet* 2, no. 7 (July 2021): 279–280. https://thelancet.com/journals/lanmic/article/PIIS2666-5247(21)00069-0/fulltext.
[163] Joe Warmington, "Opposition shockingly silent on PM's hatred of unvaccinated Canadians," *Toronto Sun*, January 6, 2022, https://torontosun.com/opinion/columnists/warmington-opposition-shockingly-silent-on-pms-hatred-of-unvaccinated-canadians.
[164] "Macron's vow to 'piss off' the unvaccinated sparks outrage," France 24, January 5, 2022, https://france24.com/en/france/20220105-macron-says-he-wants-to-piss-off-france-s-unvaccinated.

[165] Robert F. Kennedy, Jr., *The Real Anthony Fauci: Bill Gates, Big Pharma, and the Global War on Democracy and Public Health* (New York: Skyhorse Publishing, 2021), https://skyhorsepublishing.com/9781510766808/the-real-anthony-fauci/.
[166] "Federal Judge Tells FDA it Must Make Public 55,000 Pages a Month of Pfizer Vaccine Data," *FDA News*, January 10, 2022, https://fdanews.com/articles/206113-federal-judge-tells-fda-it-must-make-public-55000-pages-a-month-of-pfizer-vaccine-data.
[167] Laurie Calhoun. "On Rape: A Crime Against Humanity." *Journal of Social Philosophy* 28, no. 1 (Spring 1997): 101–109. https://onlinelibrary.wiley.com/doi/abs/10.1111/j.1467-9833.1997.tb00366.x.
[168] Laurie Calhoun, "From GITMO to the 'Killing Machine,'" January 18, 2022, https://libertarianinstitute.org/articles/from-gitmo-to-the-killing-machine/.
[169] Laurie Calhoun, "'We Murdered Some Folks': How Self-Styled Drone Warrior U.S. President Barack Obama Normalized War Crimes (Part 3)," The Drone Age, July 11, 2016, https://thedroneage.wordpress.com/2016/07/11/we-murdered-some-folks-how-self-styled-drone-warrior-us-president-barack-obama-normalized-war-crimes-part-3/.
[170] "Ensuring Patient Access and Effective Drug Enforcement Act, H.R. 4709," United States Congress (2014), https://congress.gov/bill/113th-congress/house-bill/4709.
[171] Scott Higham and Lenny Bernstein, "Who is Joe Rannazzisi: The DEA man who fought the drug companies and lost," *Washington Post*, October 15, 2017, https://washingtonpost.com/investigations/who-is-joe-rannazzisi-the-dea-man-who-fought-the-drug-companies-and-lost/2017/10/15/c3ac4b0e-b02e-11e7-be94-fabb0f1e9ffb_story.html.
[172] Laurie Calhoun, "Lessons from Fentanyl," February 16, 2022, https://libertarianinstitute.org/articles/lessons-from-fentanyl/.
[173] German Lopez, "Congress just passed a big bill to fight the opioid epidemic. But there's a catch," *Vox*, July 14, 2016, https://vox.com/2016/7/6/12101476/obama-congress-opioids-heroin.
[174] Soo Youn, "Suboxone maker Reckitt Benckiser to pay $1.4 billion in largest opioid settlement in U.S. history," ABC News, July 12, 2019, https://abcnews.go.com/Business/suboxone-maker-reckitt-benckiser-pay-14-billion-largest/story?id=64274260.
[175] "Immunization: The Basics" (Archive link), Centers for Disease Control and Prevention, http://web.archive.org/web/20210826113846/https://cdc.gov/vaccines/vac-gen/imz-basics.htm. Last modified May 17, 2018.
[176] "Immunization: The Basics." Centers for Disease Control and Prevention, https://cdc.gov/vaccines/vac-gen/imz-basics.htm. Accessed March 28, 2022.
[177] Laurie Calhoun, "It's Official: David Cameron Is Now Barack Obama's Poodle," The Drone Age, September 11, 2015, https://thedroneage.wordpress.com/2015/09/11/its-official-david-cameron-is-now-barack-obamas-poodle/.
[178] Laurie Calhoun, "Remembering the Magna Carta," The Drone Age, May 15, 2016, https://thedroneage.wordpress.com/2016/05/15/remembering-the-magna-carta/.

[179] Philip Caldwell, "Taxpayers Pony Up to Give All House Staff Peloton Memberships," *Washington Free Beacon*, May 13, 2022, https://freebeacon.com/politics/taxpayers-pony-up-to-give-all-house-staff-peloton-memberships/.
[180] "Nina Jankowicz—Mary Poppins (Disinformation Song)," YouTube video, May 10, 2022 (originally posted by Jankowicz on TikTok, February 17, 2021), https://youtube.com/watch?v=lNcEVYq2qUg.
[181] Kyle Morris, "Psaki defends Nina Jankowicz, claims DHS 'disinformation' board continuation of work under Trump," Fox News, April 29, 2022, https://foxnews.com/politics/psaki-defends-nina-jankowicz-claims-dhs-disinformation-board-continuation-work-under-trump.
[182] Ian Schwartz, "Psaki Defends DHS Panel to 'Prevent' Disinformation: 'I'm not sure who opposes that,'" Real Clear Politics, April 28, 2022, https://realclearpolitics.com/video/2022/04/28/psaki_defends_dhs_panel_to_prevent_disinformation_im_not_sure_who_opposes_that.html.
[183] "Additional Ukraine Supplemental Appropriations Act," United States Congress (2022), https://appropriations.house.gov/sites/democrats.appropriations.house.gov/files/Additional%20Ukraine%20Suplemental%20Appropriations%20Act%20Summary.pdf.
[184] "Smith-Mundt Modernization Act, H.R. 5736," United States Congress (2012), https://congress.gov/bill/112th-congress/house-bill/5736.
[185] Malou Innocent, "The Pentagon Propaganda Machine Rears Its Head," February 24, 2011, https://cato.org/blog/pentagon-propaganda-machine-rears-its-head.
[186] Julia Kollewe, "Pfizer accused of pandemic profiteering as profits double," *The Guardian*, February 8, 2022, https://theguardian.com/business/2022/feb/08/pfizer-covid-vaccine-pill-profits-sales.
[187] Zachary Evans, "New DHS Disinformation Head Dismissed Hunter Biden Emails as 'Trump Campaign Product,'" *National Review*, April 28, 2022, https://nationalreview.com/news/new-dhs-disinformation-head-dismissed-hunter-biden-emails-as-trump-campaign-product/.
[188] Laurie Calhoun, "America's Exceptional Amnesia (About Those War Criminals...)" April 13, 2022, https://libertarianinstitute.org/articles/americas-exceptional-amnesia-about-those-war-criminals/.
[189] Alex Durante, "U.S. Fiscal Response to COVID-19 Among Largest of Industrialized Countries," Tax Foundation, January 4, 2022, https://taxfoundation.org/us-covid19-fiscal-response/.
[190] "Coronavirus Country Profiles," Our World in Data, https://ourworldindata.org/coronavirus#coronavirus-country-profiles.
[191] "WISQARS Leading Causes of Death Visualization Tool," Centers for Disease Control and Prevention (CDC), https://wisqars.cdc.gov/data/lcd/home.

[192] Giacomo Tognini, "Moderna CEO Stéphane Bancel Becomes a Billionaire as Stock Jumps on Coronavirus Vaccine News," *Forbes*, April 3, 2020, https://forbes.com/sites/giacomotognini/2020/04/03/moderna-ceo-stphane-bancel-becomes-a-billionaire-as-stock-jumps-on-coronavirus-vaccine-news/?sh=71dff8bc5bf3.
[193] Aria Bendix, "The original coronavirus strain has almost disappeared in the US. One chart shows how variants took over," *Business Insider*, June 30, 2021, https://businessinsider.com/original-coronavirus-strain-replaced-by-variants-us-chart-2021-6?op=1.
[194] Michael Specter, "How Anthony Fauci Became America's Doctor," *The New Yorker*, April 10, 2020, https://newyorker.com/magazine/2020/04/20/how-anthony-fauci-became-americas-doctor.
[195] Piero Olliaro, Els Torreele, and Michel Vaillant. "COVID-19 Vaccine Efficacy and Effectiveness — The Elephant (Not) in the Room." *The Lancet* 2, no. 7 (July 2021): 279–280. https://thelancet.com/journals/lanmic/article/PIIS2666-5247(21)00069-0/fulltext.
[196] Anna Allen, "D.C. Mayor Bans Unvaccinated Children from Attending School," *Washington Free Beacon*, August 26, 2022, https://freebeacon.com/campus/dc-mayor-bans-unvaccinated-children-from-attending-school/.
[197] Salynn Boyles, "VAERS Data Confirm Myocarditis Risk After mRNA Vaccine," *Physicians Weekly*, January 27, 2022, https://physiciansweekly.com/vaers-data-confirm-myocarditis-risk-after-mrna-vaccine/.
[198] "Requirement for Proof of COVID-19 Vaccination for Air Passengers," Centers for Disease Control and Prevention, July 14, 2022, https://cdc.gov/coronavirus/2019-ncov/travelers/proof-of-vaccination.html.
[199] Robby Soave, "Anthony Fauci Says His Critics Are Attacking Science Itself," *Reason*, June 9, 2021, https://reason.com/2021/06/09/anthony-fauci-science-critics-COVID-19-chuck-todd/.
[200] Aria Bendix, "The original coronavirus strain has almost disappeared in the US. One chart shows how variants took over," *Business Insider*, June 30, 2021, https://businessinsider.com/original-coronavirus-strain-replaced-by-variants-us-chart-2021-6?op=1.
[201] Piero Olliaro, Els Torreele, and Michel Vaillant. "COVID-19 Vaccine Efficacy and Effectiveness — The Elephant (Not) in the Room." *The Lancet* 2, no. 7 (July 2021): 279–280. https://thelancet.com/journals/lanmic/article/PIIS2666-5247(21)00069-0/fulltext.
[202] Tiana Lowe, "NIH admits Fauci lied about funding Wuhan gain-of-function experiments," *Washington Examiner*, October 20, 2021, https://washingtonexaminer.com/opinion/nih-admits-fauci-lied-about-funding-wuhan-gain-of-function-experiments.
[203] Steven Quay, and Richard Muller, "The Science Suggests a Wuhan Lab Leak," *Wall Street Journal*, June 6, 2021, https://wsj.com/articles/the-science-suggests-a-wuhan-lab-leak-11622995184.

[204] Alexandre O Gérard, Audrey Laurain, Audrey Fresse, Nadège Parassol, Marine Muzzone, Fanny Rocher, Vincent L M Esnault, and Milou-Daniel Drici. "Remdesivir and Acute Renal Failure: A Potential Safety Signal From Disproportionality Analysis of the WHO Safety Database." *Clinical Pharmacology & Therapeutics* 109, no. 4 (April 2021): 1021–1024. https://pubmed.ncbi.nlm.nih.gov/33340409/.
[205] JV Chamary, "The Strange Story of Remdesivir, A Covid Drug That Doesn't Work," *Forbes*, January 31, 2021, https://forbes.com/sites/jvchamary/2021/01/31/remdesivir-covid-coronavirus/?sh=18e082fd66c2.
[206] "Drug Overdose Deaths in the U.S. Top 100,000 Annually," National Center for Health Statistics, Centers for Disease Control and Prevention, November 17, 2021, https://cdc.gov/nchs/pressroom/nchs_press_releases/2021/20211117.htm.
[207] Laurie Calhoun, "Lessons from Fentanyl," February 16, 2022, https://libertarianinstitute.org/articles/lessons-from-fentanyl/.
[208] Alex Gibney, *The Crime of the Century*, HBO Films, 2021, https://hbo.com/the-crime-of-the-century.
[209] Hunter Voegele and Ander Ugalde. "What's in the Inflation Reduction Act?" *National Law Review* 12, no. 236 (September 2022). https://natlawreview.com/article/what-s-inflation-reduction-act.
[210] "Assault Weapons Ban, H.R. 1808," United States Congress (2022), https://congress.gov/bill/117th-congress/house-bill/1808.
[211] "U.S. National Debt Clock," USDebtClock.org, https://usdebtclock.org/.
[212] Alex Gibney, *The Crime of the Century*, HBO Films, 2021, https://hbo.com/the-crime-of-the-century.
[213] Ben Westhoff, *Fentanyl, Inc.: How Rogue Chemists Are Creating the Deadliest Wave of the Opioid Epidemic* (New York: Grove Press, 2019), https://benwesthoff.com/fentanyl-inc.
[214] Christina Wilkie and Amanda Macias, "Biden says Nord Stream 2 won't go forward if Russia invades Ukraine," CNBC, February 7, 2022, https://cnbc.com/2022/02/07/biden-says-nord-stream-2-wont-go-forward-if-russia-invades-ukraine-.html.
[215] Scott Horton, *Enough Already: Time to End the War on Terrorism* (Austin: The Libertarian Institute, 2021), https://libertarianinstitute.org/books/enough-already-time-to-end-the-war-on-terrorism/.
[216] Scott Pelley, "President Joe Biden: The 2022 *60 Minutes* Interview," CBS News, September 18, 2022, https://cbsnews.com/news/president-joe-biden-60-minutes-interview-transcript-2022-09-18/.
[217] "G20 Bali Leaders' Declaration," November 16, 2022, https://whitehouse.gov/briefing-room/statements-releases/2022/11/16/g20-bali-leaders-declaration/.
[218] Kevin Liptak and Donald Judd, "President Joe Biden tests positive for COVID-19 again," *CNN Politics*, July 30, 2022, https://cnn.com/2022/07/30/politics/joe-biden-COVID-19-positive/index.html.
[219] "Obeying Orders," *Facing History*, August 11, 2017, https://facinghistory.org/resource-library/obeying-orders.

[220] Piero Olliaro, Els Torreele, and Michel Vaillant. "COVID-19 Vaccine Efficacy and Effectiveness — The Elephant (Not) in the Room." *The Lancet* 2, no. 7 (July 2021): 279–280. https://thelancet.com/journals/lanmic/article/PIIS2666-5247(21)00069-0/fulltext.
[221] Dillon Burroughs, "21 Republican Governors Join Letter Opposing Military Covid Vaccine Mandate," *The Daily Wire*, November 30, 2022, https://dailywire.com/news/21-republican-governors-join-letter-opposing-military-covid-vaccine-mandate.
[222] Leo Shane III and Jonathan Lehrfeld, "Biden signs burn pit exposure health bill into law," *Military Times*, August 10, 2022, https://militarytimes.com/veterans/2022/08/10/biden-signs-burn-pit-exposure-health-care-bill-into-law/.
[223] Maegan Vazquez, "Biden signs vital $858 billion defense bill into law, nixing military's COVID-19 vaccine mandate," *CNN Politics*, December 23, 2022, https://cnn.com/2022/12/23/politics/biden-signs-ndaa/index.html.
[224] Kaia Hubbard, "White House: Repealing Military Vaccine Mandate Would be a 'Mistake,'" *U.S. News & World Report*, December 7, 2022, https://usnews.com/news/politics/articles/2022-12-07/white-house-repealing-military-vaccine-mandate-would-be-a-mistake.
[225] "MEMORANDUM FOR SENIOR PENTAGON LEADERSHIP, COMMANDERS OF THE COMBATANT COMMANDS, DEFENSE AGENCY, AND DOD FIELD ACTIVITY DIRECTORS | Subject: Recission of August 24, 2021 and November 30, 2021 Coronavirus Disease 2019 Vaccination Requirements for Members of the Armed Forces," January 10, 2023, https://media.defense.gov/2023/Jan/10/2003143118/-1/-1/1/SECRETARY-OF-DEFENSE-MEMO-ON-RESCISSION-OF-CORONAVIRUS-DISEASE-2019-VACCINATION-REQUIREMENTS-FOR-MEMBERS-OF-THE-ARMED-FORCES.PDF.
[226] Joseph Biden, "Remarks by President Biden After Meeting with the COVID-19 Response Team," December 16, 2021, https://whitehouse.gov/briefing-room/speeches-remarks/2021/12/16/remarks-by-president-biden-after-meeting-with-members-of-the-COVID-19-response-team/.
[227] *National Federation of Independent Business v. OSHA* (21A244) and *Ohio, et al. Applicants v. OSHA* (21A247), Supreme Court of the United States (*per curiam*) (January 13, 2022.), https://supremecourt.gov/opinions/21pdf/21a244_hgci.pdf.
[228] *Biden v. Missouri* (21A240) and *HHS v. Louisiana* (21A241), Supreme Court of the United States (*per curiam*) (January 13, 2022.), https://supremecourt.gov/opinions/21pdf/21a240_d18e.pdf.
[229] "User Clip: Dr. Fauci: Best Vaccination Is Infection," C-SPAN, October 11, 2004, https://c-span.org/video/?c5009217/user-clip-dr-fauci-vaccination-infection.
[230] Spencer Kimball, "Biden administration makes at-home Covid tests available for free again this winter," CNBC, December 15, 2022, https://cnbc.com/2022/12/15/biden-admin-free-covid-home-tests.html.

[231] Connor Boyd, "America quietly extends Covid vaccination entry requirement for travels until APRIL — making U.S. an international outlier," *Daily Mail*, January 4, 2023, https://dailymail.co.uk/health/article-11600173/US-extends-Covid-vaccination-entry-requirement-travelers-APRIL.html.
[232] "International Travel Restrictions by Country," Kayak, https://kayak.com/travel-restrictions. Accessed January 17, 2023.
[233] Lee Harding, "Harms Caused by the COVID Vaccine," Frontier Centre for Public Policy (FCPP), February 12, 2023, https://fcpp.org/2023/02/12/harms-caused-by-the-covid-vaccine/.
[234] Tarun Sai Lomte, "The safety profile and the actual known adverse effects of the COVID-19 vaccines in at-risk and healthy individuals," *Medical News*, February 7, 2023, https://news-medical.net/news/20230207/The-safety-profile-and-the-actual-known-adverse-effects-of-COVID-19-vaccines-in-at-risk-and-healthy-individuals.aspx.
[235] Jennifer Couzin-Frankel, "Thousands report unusual menstruation cycles after COVID-19 vaccination," *Science*, July 15, 2022, https://science.org/content/article/thousands-report-unusual-menstruation-patterns-after-COVID-19-vaccination.
[236] "Pfizer Director Jordon Trishton Walker Shares Concern for COVID Vaccine Effect on Women's Reproductive Health," Project Veritas, February 2, 2023, https://projectveritas.com/news/new-pfizer-director-jordon-trishton-walker-shares-concern-for-covid-vaccine/.
[237] Snigdha Prakash and Vikki Valentine, "Timeline: The Rise and Fall of Vioxx," NPR, November 10, 2007, https://npr.org/2007/11/10/5470430/timeline-the-rise-and-fall-of-vioxx.
[238] Florencia Halperin, MD, "Weight-loss drug Belviq recalled," *Harvard Health Blog*, April 9, 2020, https://health.harvard.edu/blog/weight-loss-drug-belviq-recalled-2020040919439.
[239] "Internal Documents: Bayer Knew of Baycol Dangers — NYT," Alliance for Human Research Protection, February 23, 2003, https://ahrp.org/internal-documents-bayer-knew-of-baycol-dangers-nyt/.
[240] Nabin K. Shrestha, Patrick C. Burke, Amy S. Nowacki, James F. Simon, Amanda Hagen, and Steven M. Gordon, "Effectiveness of the Coronavirus Disease 2019 (COVID-19) Bivalent Vaccine," medRxiv, December 19, 2022, https://medrxiv.org/content/10.1101/2022.12.17.22283625v1.full.pdf.
[241] "Recommended Vaccinations for Infants and Children, Parent-Friendly Version: Birth through 6 Years, United States, 2023," Centers for Disease Control and Prevention, February 10, 2023, https://cdc.gov/vaccines/schedules/easy-to-read/child-easyread.html.
[242] Piero Olliaro, Els Torreele, and Michel Vaillant. "COVID-19 Vaccine Efficacy and Effectiveness — The Elephant (Not) in the Room." *The Lancet* 2, no. 7 (July 2021): 279–280. https://thelancet.com/journals/lanmic/article/PIIS2666-5247(21)00069-0/fulltext.
[243] Nabin K. Shrestha, Patrick C. Burke, Amy S. Nowacki, James F. Simon, Amanda Hagen, and Steven M. Gordon, "Effectiveness of the Coronavirus Disease 2019 (COVID-19) Bivalent Vaccine," medRxiv, December 19, 2022, https://medrxiv.org/content/10.1101/2022.12.17.22283625v1.full.pdf.

[244] Stephen Chen, "Coronavirus mutation could threaten the race to develop vaccine," *South China Morning Post*, April 14, 2020, https://scmp.com/news/china/science/article/3079678/coronavirus-mutation-threatens-race-develop-vaccine.
[245] David M. Morens, Jeffery K. Taubenberger, and Anthony S. Fauci. "Rethinking next-generation vaccines for coronaviruses, influenzaviruses, and other respiratory viruses." *Cell Host & Microbe* 31, no. 1 (January 2023): 146–157. https://ncbi.nlm.nih.gov/pmc/articles/PMC9832587/.
[246] "WMA Declaration of Helsinki — Ethical Principles for Medical Research Involving Human Subjects." World Medical Association. September 6, 2022. https://wma.net/policies-post/wma-declaration-of-helsinki-ethical-principles-for-medical-research-involving-human-subjects/.
[247] Derek Thompson, "The Pandemic's Wrongest Man," *The Atlantic*, April 1, 2021, https://theatlantic.com/ideas/archive/2021/04/pandemics-wrongest-man/618475/.
[248] Alex Berenson, "Berenson v. Biden is coming…" *Unreported Truths*, January 27, 2023, https://alexberenson.substack.com/p/berenson-v-biden-is-coming.
[249] Robby Soave, "Anthony Fauci Says His Critics Are Attacking Science Itself," *Reason*, June 9, 2021, https://reason.com/2021/06/09/anthony-fauci-science-critics-COVID-19-chuck-todd/.
[250] Steve Bannon, "Bannon's War Room: Dr. Malone Reveals Study by Fauci Admitting mRNA Vaccines Hardly Work," Rumble video, February 9, 2023, https://rumble.com/v28wfde-dr.-malone-reveals-study-by-fauci-admitting-mrna-vaccines-hardly-work.html.
[251] Robert F. Kennedy, Jr., *The Real Anthony Fauci: Bill Gates, Big Pharma, and the Global War on Democracy and Public Health* (New York: Skyhorse Publishing, 2021), https://skyhorsepublishing.com/9781510766808/the-real-anthony-fauci/.
[252] Natalie Rahhal, "Pfizer CEO 'not certain' its Covid vaccine prevents transmission," *Daily Mail*, December 4, 2020, https://dailymail.co.uk/health/article-9018547/Pfizer-CEO-not-certain-covid-shot-prevents-transmission.html.
[253] "Pfizer and BioNTech Announce Vaccine Candidate Against COVID-19 Achieved Success in First Interim Analysis from Phase 3 Study," November 9, 2020, https://pfizer.com/news/press-release/press-release-detail/pfizer-and-biontech-announce-vaccine-candidate-against.
[254] "Fact Check: Preventing transmission never required for COVID vaccines' initial approval; Pfizer vax did reduce transmission of early variants," Reuters, October 14, 2022, https://reuters.com/article/factcheck-pfizer-vaccine-transmission/fact-check-preventing-transmission-never-required-for-covid-vaccines-initial-approval-pfizer-vax-did-reduce-transmission-of-early-variants-idUSL1N31F20E.
[255] "Immunization: The Basics." Accessed March 14, 2023.
[256] Alex Gibney, *The Crime of the Century*, HBO Films, 2021, https://hbo.com/the-crime-of-the-century.

[257] Ravi Chandra, MD, DFAPA, "Calling COVID-19 a 'Chinese Virus' or 'Kung Flu' is Racist," *Psychology Today*, March 18, 2020, https://psychologytoday.com/us/blog/the-pacific-heart/202003/calling-COVID-19-chinese-virus-or-kung-flu-is-racist.
[258] Louis Casiano, "Biden signs COVID declassification bill, hints at withholding some information," Fox News, March 20, 2023, https://foxnews.com/politics/biden-signs-covid-declassification-bill-hints-withholding-some-information.
[259] Stephen Collinson, Caitlin Hu, and Shelby Rose, "'No more feebleness': Pelosi in showdown with Beijing over potential Taiwan visit," *CNN Politics*, July 26, 2022, https://cnn.com/2022/07/26/politics/nancy-pelosi-taiwan-visit-showdown/index.html.
[260] "Protecting Speech from Government Interference Act, H.R. 140," United States Congress (2023), https://congress.gov/bill/118th-congress/house-bill/140.
[261] Peter Kasperowicz, "Democrat blocks GOP bill to end Biden's vaccine requirement for non-US travelers," Fox News, March 22, 2023, https://foxnews.com/politics/democrat-blocks-gop-bill-end-bidens-vaccine-requirement-non-us-travelers.
[262] Margot Cleveland, "The Censorship Complex Isn't a 'Tinfoil Hat' Conspiracy, and the 'Twitter Files' Just Dropped More Proof," *The Federalist*, March 10, 2023, https://thefederalist.com/2023/03/10/the-censorship-complex-isnt-a-tinfoil-hat-conspiracy-and-the-twitter-files-just-dropped-more-proof/.
[263] Nomia Iqbal and Sam Cabral, "COVID-19 origin debate 'squashed,' ex-CDC chief Dr Robert Redfield claims," BBC News, March 9, 2023, https://bbc.com/news/world-us-canada-64891745.
[264] Katherine J. Wu, "The Strongest Evidence Yet That an Animal Started the Pandemic," *The Atlantic*, March 16, 2023, https://theatlantic.com/science/archive/2023/03/covid-origins-research-raccoon-dogs-wuhan-market-lab-leak/673390/.
[265] "BREAKING: Confidential Pfizer Documents Reveal Pharmaceutical Giant Had 'Evidence' Suggesting 'Increased Risk of Myocarditis' Following COVID-19 Vaccinations in Early 2022," Project Veritas, March 16, 2023, https://projectveritas.com/news/breaking-confidential-pfizer-documents-reveal-pharmaceutical-giant-had/.
[266] David Edwards, "Rand Paul stunned by Moderna CEO: Less risk of myocarditis for people who take vaccine," MSN, March 22, 2023, https://msn.com/en-us/health/medical/rand-paul-stunned-by-moderna-ceo-less-risk-of-myocarditis-for-people-who-take-vaccine/ar-AA18WPyH.
[267] Beth Mole, "As COVID vaccine patent dispute drags on, Moderna forks over $400M to NIH," Ars Technica, February 24, 2023, https://arstechnica.com/science/2023/02/moderna-forks-over-400m-to-nih-amid-dispute-over-covid-vaccine-ip/.
[268] Spencer Kimball, "Watch: Moderna CEO Stéphane Bancel testifies before Senate on Covid vaccine price hike," CNBC, March 22, 2023, https://cnbc.com/2023/03/22/watch-live-moderna-ceo-stephane-bancel-testifies-before-senate-on-covid-vaccine-price-hike.html.

Index of Names and Places Cited

Selected Praise for Laurie Calhoun's Other Works

We Kill Because We Can: From Soldiering to Assassination in the Drone Age

"Vital and compelling reading."

– Counterfire

"Fresh, well-researched and well-written… provides an occasion to think about the deep implications of killing people through drones."

– openDemocracy

"This timely book… has exposed the ethical and moral bankruptcy and shortsighted objectives of the Predator drone programme."

– *Pacific Journalism Review*

"Targeted assassination through the use of Predator drones has become the most dramatic military novelty of the twenty-first century. Laurie Calhoun's brilliant enquiry into the mindset of its perpetrators and supporters is a chilling reminder of how far we have strayed from the concept of 'a just war.'"

– Richard Gott,
author of *Britain's Empire: Resistance, Rebellion and Revolt*

"A comprehensive and shocking survey of the dirty consequences of U.S. drone strikes. Calhoun provides important information on civilian casualties, which puts the lie to the CIA's denial of such losses. This important work will be helpful in any re-examination of drone policy."

– Melvin A. Goodman, former CIA analyst
and author of *National Insecurity: The Cost of American Militarism*

"The drone assassination campaign is the most extraordinary global terror campaign yet conceived and executed. This chilling and comprehensive survey more than amply demonstrates that drone strikes are war crimes, and that this new technology is not only an effective device of mass murder at a distance, but that it also eliminates barriers for commanders to 'prosecute wars at their caprice.' That the technology will sooner or later be directed against the perpetrators is hardly in doubt, as the cycle of violence takes its predictable course."

– *Noam Chomsky*

"By far the best book on drone warfare and the ethics of targeted assassinations to date. Powerful and eloquent, Laurie Calhoun elucidates a set of convincing arguments as to why drone killing is ethically indefensible and strategically counterproductive, but also why it is so seductive to our governments. It should be required reading for politicians, military planners and journalists."

– Richard Jackson,
author of *Confessions of a Terrorist*

"In *We Kill Because We Can*, Laurie Calhoun poses worrisome questions that our government should be forced to answer, such as how an unarmed person can pose an imminent threat, and whether drones have inspired more terrorist attacks than they have prevented. Calhoun also makes some very searing but well-reasoned analogies between our government and the mafia; Bush, Obama and bin Laden; and targeted killings as simply assassinations. The book forces the reader to question our government's policies in terms of efficacy, adherence to law, and, most painfully, moral grounds. It is a clarion call to reverse course if we ever want to see an end to our military adventures abroad and what the author refers to as our 'single-minded obsession with lethality as a solution to conflict.' Read it and act!"

– Medea Benjamin, co-founder of CODEPINK for Peace
and author of *Drone Warfare: Killing by Remote Control*

War and Delusion: A Critical Examination

"This work is timeless and timely. It is timely because it helps shed light on our understanding of contemporary wars beyond the just war paradigm; it is timeless because the critique is well crafted and substantive [enough] to endure the test of time. The author manages to demolish the just war paradigm brick by brick all the way down to its very foundation… She exposes its emptiness for all to see and pushes students of war to seek new and better understandings of why we go to war and how we should conduct wars in the twenty-first century."

– Ajume H. Wingo,
Director of the Center for Values and Social Policy,
Associate Professor at the University of Colorado at Boulder,
and author of *Veil Politics in Liberal Democratic States*

"Laurie Calhoun provides a passionate, provocative, challenging and inspiring critique of the war ideology. She uncovers the rhetoric behind the justification for the use of violence, and shows how powerful and pervasive is the machine designed to criminalize opponents. It is well known that these methods of propaganda have been widely used by totalitarian regimes, but this book confirms that liberal democracies are equally using them and that the populace is unaware and manipulated. To unmask this ideological apparatus is a fundamental precondition to sustain the hope of making war obsolete as a method to sort out controversies."

– Daniele Archibugi,
Italian National Research Council, Rome,
Birkbeck College, University of London,
and author of *The Global Commonwealth of Citizens: Toward Cosmopolitan Democracy*

Philosophy Unmasked: A Skeptic's Critique

"A bracing gale of fresh thinking about the meaning and significance of philosophy. Calhoun's subject is both the idea of philosophy itself and what has become of it in the academic setting. It is at once argumentative performance, metaphilosophical reflection, and razor-sharp critique of the academic status quo in philosophy today. Calhoun is the most consistent and unsettling skeptic I have read. This book is hard-hitting and controversial, but also well and carefully written, and cannot be read with indifference by anyone who cares about philosophy."

– Barry Allen,
author of *Truth in Philosophy*

"Excellent and extraordinary. Calhoun's root idea — that at bottom philosophy is a matter of seduction — is, to put it mildly, disturbing to most philosophers. Her critique will not be read with indifference by them or by those in other academic areas where there are 'experts' and 'acolytes.'"

– James Kellenberger, author of *Relationship Morality*

"A provocative statement of analytic philosophy's current discontents."

– Babette E. Babich,
author of *Nietzsche's Philosophy of Science*

Also by Laurie Calhoun

Theodicy: A Metaphilosophical Investigation

You Can Leave: a novel

Laminated Souls: a novel

The Libertarian Institute

Check out the Libertarian Institute at libertarianinstitute.org. It's Scott Horton, Sheldon Richman, Laurie Calhoun, James Bovard, Kyle Anzalone, Keith Knight and the best libertarian writers and podcast hosts on the Internet. We are a 501(c)(3) tax-exempt charitable organization. EIN 83-2869616.

Regular donors of $5 or more per month by way of Patreon or Paypal get access to the /r/scotthortonshow group on Reddit.com. Info at scotthorton.org/donate.

Help support our efforts — including our project to purchase wholesale copies of this book to send to important congressmen and women, antiwar groups and influential people in the media. We don't have a big marketing department to push this effort. We need your help to do it. And thank you.

libertarianinstitute.org/donate or
The Libertarian Institute
612 W. 34th St.
Austin, TX 78705

Check out all of our other great Libertarian Institute books at libertarianinstitute.org/books:

Hotter Than the Sun: Time to Abolish Nuclear Weapons by Scott Horton
Enough Already: Time to End the War on Terrorism by Scott Horton
Fool's Errand: Time to End the War in Afghanistan by Scott Horton
Voluntaryist Handbook by Keith Knight
The Great Ron Paul: The Scott Horton Show Interviews 2004–2019
No Quarter: The Ravings of William Norman Grigg, edited by Tom Eddlem
Coming to Palestine by Sheldon Richman
What Social Animals Owe to Each Other by Sheldon Richman

Keep a look out for more great titles to be published in 2023.

Made in the USA
Columbia, SC
25 October 2023

24952295R00159